Overcoming Arthritis

See How Holistic Treatments Can
Cure Arthritis, Fibromyalgia,
Chronic Fatigue Syndrome and
Other Conditions

OVERCOMING

ARTHRITIS

Using The Following Therapies:

- •Natural Hormones
- •Vitamins and Minerals
- •Allergy Elimination

- •Detoxification
- •Diet
- •Water

•And More!!

David Brownstein, M.D.

Foreword by Jonathan Wright, M.D.

For further copies of <u>Overcoming Arthritis:</u>

Call **(888) 647-5616** or send a check or money order for $20.00 ($15.00 + $5.00 S+H) or for Michigan residents $20.90 ($15.00 + $5.00 S&H + $.90 sales tax) to:

> Medical Alternatives Press
> 4173 Fieldbrook Rd.
> West Bloomfield, MI 48323

Or, visit our website at: **www.drbrownstein.com**

ISBN: 978-0-9660882-1-2

Medical Alternatives Press
4173 Fieldbrook Rd.
West Bloomfield, MI 48323
(888) 647-5616
www.drbrownstein.com

Acknowledgements

I gratefully acknowledge the help I have received from my friends and colleagues. They have tirelessly read and re-read the manuscript. Without their support, this book would not have been possible.

I would also like to thank my staff for all of their hard work and dedication. I truly appreciate all of your comments as this manuscript was being written.

To the editors, my enduring gratitude. My wife Allison, my parents Ruth and Ellis Brownstein, my sisters, Linda Laird and Leslie Rosenwasser, my mother-in-law and father in-law, Shirley and Phil Selko, my sister-in-law Adrienne Selko, Martha Minano (for reading and re-reading and re-reading again), Kristin Babcock, F. Batmanghelidj, M.D., Harry Eidenier, Jr., Ph.D., Rick Ng, M.D., Jeffrey Nusbaum, M.D., Robert Radtke, D.C., and Jonathan Wright, M.D.

About The Author

David Brownstein, M.D. is a Board-Certified Family Physician who utilizes the best of conventional and alternative therapies. He is the medical director for the Center for Holistic Medicine in West Bloomfield, MI. Dr. Brownstein is a Clinical Assistant Professor of Internal Medicine at Wayne State University School of Medicine. Dr. Brownstein is board-certified by the American Academy of Family Physicians. He is a member of the American College for the Advancement in Medicine (ACAM), American Academy of Preventive Medicine and the American Academy of Family Physicians.

A WORD OF CAUTION TO THE READER

The information presented in this book is based on the training and professional experience of the author. The treatments recommended in this book should not be undertaken without first consulting a physician. Proper laboratory and clinical monitoring is essential to achieving the goals of finding safe and natural treatments. This book was written for informational and educational purposes only. It is not intended to be used as medical advice.

To my family, my past, present and future
Allison, Hailey, Jessica. All my love.

And,

To my patients. Without your stories, none of this would be
possible. I learn from you every single day and I cannot thank you
enough.

What Others Are Saying About
Overcoming Arthritis

"The cardinal distinctions of a present day healer, apart from any formal training in modern medicine, are an open and receptive scientific mind and unselfish caring for the suffering sick in need of help. Dr. Brownstein, endowed with these qualities, and armed with the first-hand experience of a new medical breakthrough, has produced this in his new book, *Overcoming Arthritis*."

>F. Batmanghelidj, M.D., Falls Church, VA
>Author, *Your Body's Many Cries for Water* and *ABC of Asthma, Allergies and Lupus.*

"This book demonstrates great insight into pioneering medicine in nutritional deficiency and chronic infection in chronic diseases. It challenges the efficacy of current clinical practice and leaves a trail for interested medical practitioners to follow."

>Kerrie Davis, Australia
>Fellow, Royal Australian College of General Practitioners,

"As a Scleroderma patient since 1982, I struggled to find a safe and effective treatment. This book provides insight and direction in such a safe and effective treatment. I recommend this book as a life-changing guide for anyone suffering with an arthritic disorder."

>Pat Ganger, Deleware, Ohio.
>Former Director, The Road Back Foundation

"Every now and then, and certainly not often enough, I have the privilege to read a book that provides clear, concise and useful information on the treatment of various conditions that often leave myself and others like me speculating why, after our best efforts, the patient has not improved. This book provides answers to a myriad of these questions concerning how the problem(s) develop and how to get best results in the shortest possible time. The book is a milestone in the treatment of difficult chronic conditions and offers hope to those ill individuals who have had no hope. In short, it is a "must read" for anyone wondering about or treating chronic illness."

Harry O. Eidenier, Jr., Ph.D.,
Director of Research for Viotron International and DSD International

"While we see hundreds of books written on arthritis, there is none like this one. Doctor Brownstein's book, _Overcoming Arthritis,_ stands out. It is unique and carries a different message: Find the underlying problem and fix it. It is a book that can help you overcome your pain and discomfort."

Devi Nambudripod, Ph.D, D.C.,L.Ac., Buena Park, CA, Founder of NAET and author of _Say Goodbye to Illness, Living Pain Free with Acupressure and Say Goodbye To...Series._

"Anybody with arthritis should read Dr. Brownstein's book, _Overcoming Arthritis_. No disease has ever been cured without understanding and addressing its cause – and Dr. Brownstein's book does just that. He offers a balanced, holistic approach to healing, based on the fast-growing body of evidence that most forms of arthritis are infectious in their etiology."

> Henry Scammell, Orleans, MA
> Author of _The New Arthritis Breakthrough_ and President,
> The Road Back Foundation

"This book, like your first, _The Miracle of Natural Hormones_ has combined complementary and orthodox medicine using a scientific basis while retaining the art of simplicity enabling all to read and understand."

> Lynnette Wright, N.D.,
> Herbalist, Nutritionist. Australia

"Dr. Brownstein uses a holistic approach to the treatment of arthritis which is based on an individualized program using nutritional support, natural hormones and detoxification. This book is an essential tool for patients and doctors alike looking for better ways to help heal arthritis, chronic fatigue and fibromyalgia."

> David M. Goldstein, M.D.
> Medical Director, North Hills Natural Medicine
> Pittsburgh, PA

Contents

Foreword

There's no disease caused by a lack of a prescription drug. Yet when we're ill enough to see a doctor, prescription drugs are often the treatment we're told to take. It's not the doctor's fault. For nearly a century, under the combined influence of the patent medicine (pharmaceutical) industry and government "authorities" (Food and Drug Administration), medical schools have told their students that non-surgical disease treatment should use molecules not naturally found in human biochemistry. Most frequently, these patent-medicine ("prescription drug") molecules are not even found naturally on our planet! (No, this isn't a plot by "space aliens": To patent a molecule, it's a *requirement* that it *not* be naturally occurring.)

Obviously, we don't become ill because we need molecules that aren't part of the normal functioning of our bodies, molecules that aren't even part of the natural world that includes the human species. The causes of illness lie elsewhere, and we should be looking for those causes. If we look hard and still can't find them, we should first try overcoming the illness (or at least achieving symptom relief) with molecules natural to our bodies or to our world. Sadly, medical students are educated to use entirely un-natural, alien, patent medicines instead.

It hasn't always been this way. Thousands of years ago, young doctors were told "first look for the cause". When the cause couldn't be found, they had only natural remedies to turn to.

The above isn't written to imply that "modern medicine" has made no progress at all. In many areas, progress has been tremendous. Surgical skills and procedures are (as far as we know) the best in human history. (Could it be more than coincidence that there's no progress stifling "Federal Surgical Procedures Administration"?) Modern emergency medicine saves lives that would have been lost in prior decades and centuries. (There's no "Federal Emergency Room Administration", either.) Yet with few exceptions non-surgical, non-emergency "mainstream medicine" continues to rely on unnatural molecules (we *do* have a federal Food and Drug Administration) and unnatural energies ("radiation therapy") which rarely cure disease, have many bad effects, and are pricing themselves beyond reach.

In what follows, Dr. David Brownstein shows us a better way, the way of natural and what some call "integrative" medicine. The approach advocated by Dr. Brownstein is a return to a more logical and conservative approach to health care. Logical, because natural medicine looks for causes and how to correct them. Logical, because most natural medicine treatment uses materials found in our bodies naturally (food, amino acids, vitamins, minerals, essential fatty acids), or materials found in nature, such as herbs, that our bodies can almost always easily metabolize.

Patent medicine (pharmaceutical) treatment is basically illogical: Would you fix your reliable old Chevrolet with Volvo parts? Why attempt to heal natural bodies with "alien" molecules?

And conservative? Hasn't "natural medicine" been termed 'risky', 'radical' or possibly 'dangerous' by "authorities" at our universities, the American Medical Association, or the Food and Drug Administration? To answer these critics, we need only read their own publications. Let's look at one of the articles in the July 26th 2000 *Journal of the American Medical Association.* It tells us that approximately 106,000 people die in hospitals every year from patent medicines! It just makes sense to try the more conservative, natural approach before using much more risky and dangerous patent medications.

As Dr. Brownstein tells us, natural medicine is more than just putting natural things into our bodies. It also involves *removing* things that don't belong, things that hinder the normal, healthy functioning of our bodies. Most of us, even medical doctors, know that removing nicotine, "tar", and carbon monoxide from our bodies will promote better health. Few doctors as yet recognize how important it also is to remove allergies, sensitivities, heavy metals such as mercury, lead, and cadmium, water contaminants such as chlorine and fluoride, and so on, as Dr. Brownstein illustrates so well.

What about the antibiotics emphasized in this book? Aren't they "conventional" medicine, prescription drugs, patent medicines? Yes and no. Like conventional patent medicines, antibiotics are available only by prescription, but nearly all are natural in origin. Remember the "first antibiotic", penicillin? It was discovered after bacteria started dying on a culture plate. The bacteria had been growing near a mold, *Penicillium*, which naturally secreted penicillin to kill the bacteria around it. From another point of view, antibiotic use might be viewed as an example of "integrative medicine", a relatively new term describing the blending the best of both "conventional" and "natural" medicine.

I hope that reading Dr. Brownstein's excellent introduction to a more natural, logical, conservative (not to mention more effective!) approach to disease treatment and prevention will stimulate you not only to follow his recommendations, but to further explore the many other aspects of natural medicine. You and your family will be much healthier if you do!

And remember…headaches aren't caused by aspirin deficiency, we don't get anxious because our brains need Valium….*there's no disease caused by lack of a prescription drug.*

Jonathan V. Wright M.D.
Medical Director, Tahoma Clinic
Kent, Washington
Lecturer and author of books that have sold over 750,000 copies
Book of Nutritional Therapy, Rodale Press, 1979
Guide to Healing with Nutrition, Rodale Press, 1984
Co-Author, *Natural Hormone Replacement for Women Over 45*, Smart Publications, 1998
Co-Author, *The Natural Pharmacy*, Prima Health, 1998

Co-Author, *Maximize Your Vitality and Potency for Men Over 40*, Smart Publications, 1999
Co-Author, *The Patient's Book of Natural Healing*, Prima Health, 1999

"The doctor of the future will give no medicine, but will interest the patient in the care of the human frame, in diet and in the cause and prevention of disease."

Thomas Edison

Chapter 1

Introduction

Introduction

Arthritis comes from the Greek words *arthron* (joint) and *itis* (inflammation). It is a broad term that can accompany many different diseases (such as rheumatoid arthritis, osteoarthritis and Lyme's disease) and can be an acute or a chronic illness. The impact of arthritis on the population is staggering.

Arthritis is one of the most prevalent conditions in medicine today. Thirty-two million Americans, almost one in eight, are affected with arthritis.[1] Estimates are that by the year 2020, sixty million Americans, or 18% of the population, will be suffering from some form of arthritis.[2] Arthritis is the leading cause of disability in the United States and results in more than five million hospitalizations per year with an estimated cost of $82 billion. The cost of arthritis in the United States has been estimated to be 1.1% of the gross national product.[3]

In conventional medicine (i.e., medicine that is commonly taught in medical schools), there is no consensus on what causes arthritis. The logical question to ponder is this: if you don't understand the cause of an illness, then how can you effectively treat the illness? Since conventional medicine does not understand the cause of many chronic illnesses (e.g., arthritis, chronic fatigue syndrome, fibromyalgia, etc.), the conventional therapies presently in use are ineffective and often toxic.

For over five decades, nonsteroidal anti-inflammatory drugs (NSAID's) have been the method of treatment for arthritic disorders. If these items fail, more powerful steroids or drugs such as chemotherapeutic agents are employed. In my experience, the results of using these drug therapies are dismal. These drugs may temporarily alleviate the symptoms in arthritic disorders, but they do little to reverse or even halt the progression of the illness. In addition, NSAID drug therapies do not provide the body with the substances it needs to heal itself. In fact, because of the toxicity of NSAID's, the opposite often occurs: these items will actually inhibit healing in the body and weaken the immune system.

Prolonged use of NSAID's is often harmful. It is estimated that 16,500 patients with rheumatoid arthritis or osteoarthritis die annually from the toxic effects of NSAID's (a total which is similar to the number of deaths from AIDS).[4] Furthermore, studies have shown that the prolonged use of NSAID's will inhibit cartilage formation in arthritic patients and actually worsen arthritic conditions. It is well known that prolonged use of steroids (in large, pharmacologic doses) and chemotherapeutic agents will suppress the immune system and make the body more susceptible to illness.

4

There is a better way to treat these chronic conditions. I have found that a holistic approach, as outlined in this book, is the most effective way to treat many chronic diseases. A holistic approach is one that uses combinations of safe, natural therapies, with or without drug therapies, to treat the underlying cause of the illness and to support the body's immune system as it recovers from the disease.

The ideas outlined in this book include a regimen of vitamins, minerals, natural hormones, water, a balanced diet and detoxification of the body. In addition, drug therapies, such as small doses of antibiotics, may be necessary to treat the infectious cause of the illness. I believe the best results are achieved when these therapies are used in combination, rather than used individually. This is in contrast to conventional medicine's ineffective approach of only using drug therapies to treat a chronic illness.

This book was written to give hope to those who suffer with arthritis. By using the holistic approach outlined in this book, you can overcome arthritis and achieve your optimum health. Related disorders, such as fibromyalgia and chronic fatigue syndrome can also be successfully treated with this program. I see the positive results with this holistic regimen every day in my medical practice.

This book contains eleven chapters describing my holistic approach to the treatment of these chronic conditions. In Chapter 2, I describe how many different arthritic disorders, as well as fibromyalgia and chronic fatigue syndrome, may have an infectious cause and how the use of small amounts of antibiotics have been shown to be very helpful in treating many of these disorders.

More than fifty years of research has shown that the mycoplasma bacteria can produce arthritis in animals that exactly mimics the arthritis in humans. Dr. Thomas Brown was a pioneer in diagnosing and treating arthritic disorders. Dr. Brown successfully treated many individuals with small amounts of antibiotics, a treatment which stopped the progression and often reversed the illness. Chapter 2 will describe Dr. Brown's work and the way in which small doses of antibiotics can be successfully introduced into a holistic program to help the body fight back and recover from arthritis.

But the story does not end there. As previously stated, I have found that combining the use of antibiotics with other therapies (that actually provide the immune system with substances to heal itself) is the most effective way to promote healing of many different chronic disorders such as arthritis, fibromyalgia and chronic fatigue syndrome. Chapter 3 will discuss how a holistic approach can effectively treat fibromyalgia and chronic fatigue syndrome.

Most individuals with a chronic illness have an imbalance in their hormonal system. Chapters 4 and 5 will explain the importance of a properly functioning hormonal system. Unless the hormonal system is properly evaluated and treated, recovering from a chronic illness can be very difficult. In addition, these chapters will describe how the use of natural hormones, (i.e., natural thyroid hormone, DHEA, natural progesterone, natural testosterone, and human growth hormone) are much more effective than the commonly prescribed synthetic agents such as Synthroid or Provera.

The "Standard American Diet" with its reliance on too many carbohydrates and the over-consumption of refined products (made primarily with refined sugar and flour) causes nutrient deficiencies and can lead to a poorly functioning immune system. An inadequate diet can set the stage for the development of a chronic illness. Furthermore, it is impossible to overcome a chronic illness without obtaining the proper nutrients from the diet. Chapter 6 will describe how a balanced diet, with adequate amounts of protein, fats and carbohydrates, can provide the body with the basic raw materials necessary to promote a healthy immune system and allow the healing process to begin.

Chapter 7 reviews the importance of treating food and environmental allergies. I have found that a large percentage of patients suffering from a chronic illness also have food and environmental allergies. Allergies can lead to nutrient depletion and can inhibit the proper functioning of the immune system. Chapter 7 will show how a safe, simple acupressure technique, Nambudripod's Allergy Elimination Technique (NAET), can be utilized to overcome allergies. I have used NAET for over six years, and I can attest to its success in eliminating allergies and helping the immune system regain its strength.

People suffering from chronic illness will not heal unless their bodies are adequately hydrated with water. Chapter 8 describes why dehydration is a major health problem in the United States and how dehydration can be a major factor in the development of a chronic illness.

Chapter 9 will discuss the relationship between vitamin and mineral deficiencies and chronic illness. Dr. Majid Ali, a pioneer in the use of natural items to treat illness, claims, "Injured tissues heal with nutrients, not with drugs."[5] This is a simple statement, but it underscores the fact that it is essential to properly evaluate all individuals who suffer from a chronic illness for nutrient imbalances. Chapter 9 provides specific recommendations on the use of supplements (i.e., vitamins, minerals and herbs) to promote healing in those who suffer from chronic illness.

Finally, detoxification of the body is a very important step in the healing process. In an industrialized society, we are exposed to a "mountain" of toxins every day. These toxins include pesticides, heavy metals and hydrocarbons. Exposure to these toxins can cause problems with the immune system, the hormonal system, the neurological system and, in fact, the entire body. I have found elevated toxin levels in many of those who suffer with a chronic illness. Chapter 10 describes how to determine whether you have elevated levels of heavy metals and how to rid your body of these dangerous toxins. In addition, Chapter 10 will help you begin a detoxification program to start you on the path to wellness.

The success I have experienced with using these holistic treatments inspired me to write this book. I am convinced that only a holistic approach, one that uses a combination of natural items that support the body, will be successful in overcoming a chronic illness. The human body has a remarkable ability to heal itself and desires to be in a state of optimum health. Remember Dr. Ali's statement: "Injured tissues heal with nutrients, not with drugs." Common sense suggests that we need to provide the body with the necessary raw materials (i.e., vitamins, minerals, herbs, natural hormones, and other natural agents) in order to begin the healing process. People do not have to suffer with their illness. There is a way to overcome chronic disease. This book will provide you with a unique holistic approach to overcoming chronic illnesses (arthritis, fibromyalgia, chronic fatigue syndrome and others) and to achieving your optimum health.

Final Thoughts

All of the information presented in this book may seem overwhelming at first. Adopting a holistic approach as outlined in this book, (including eating a healthy diet, drinking adequate amounts of water, etc.,) can help you recover from arthritis, fibromyalgia, chronic fatigue syndrome and other illnesses. You can overcome a chronic illness. Don't be overwhelmed by the information in this book. Take it step by step and you will begin to see positive results.

[1] Praemer, A, et al. Musculoskeletal conditions in the United States. 2nd ed. Rosemeont, Il: American Academy of Orthopedic Surgeons, 1999

[2] DiNubile, Nicholas. "Osteoarthritis of the Knee, a Special Report." The Physician and Sportsmedicine, May, 2000

[3] DiNubile, Nicholas. IBID.

[4] Wolf, MM, et al. "Gastrointestinal toxicity of nonsteroidal anti-inflammatory drugs." NEJM. 1999; 340:1888

[5] Ali, Majid. Preface to The Miracle of Natural Hormones, 2nd Edition, by David Brownstein. Medical Alternatives Press, 1999.

Chapter 2

The Arthritis-Infection Connection

The Arthritis-Infection Connection

Table 1: Diseases That May Have An Underlying Infectious Etiology

Rheumatoid Arthritis	Polymyalgia Rheumatica
Scleroderma	Polymyositis
Fibromyalgia	Psoriatic Arthritis
Chronic Fatigue Syndrome	Juvenile Arthritis
Gulf War Syndrome	Sjogren's Syndrome
Vasculitis	Lupus
Reiter's Syndrome	Multiple Sclerosis
Hashimoto's Thyroiditis	Crohn's Disease
Graves' Disease	Ulcerative Colitis

In order to effectively treat an illness, one must understand the cause of the illness. Sadly, conventional treatments for arthritis (i.e., anti-inflammatory drugs or disease modifying drugs) do not address the cause; they only treat the symptoms of illness. Perhaps an infectious process **is the cause** of the disorders listed in Table 1. Table 1 lists some of the diseases that are proposed to have an infectious etiology and that may respond to antibiotic therapy.

The search for a bacterial cause for certain types of arthritis has been ongoing for over fifty years. There are numerous bacteria, viruses and fungi that have been implicated in various forms of arthritis (See Table 2.)   A bacterium known as mycoplasma has been suggested as a causative factor in arthritis for well over fifty years. Mycoplasma was first isolated in humans by Dr. Louis Dienes in 1932. Dr. Albert Sabin was able to isolate mycoplasma in arthritic mice in 1938.[1]

Table 2: Infectious Causes of Arthritis

Staphylococcus aureus	Chlamydia
Streptococcus	Brucella
Neisseria	Coxiella
Candida	Mycoplasma
Mycobacterium tuberculosis	Hepatitis B
Borrelia burgdorferi	Parvovirus B19
Treponema pallidum	HIV
Fungi	Rickettsia

In 1939, Dr. Thomas McPherson Brown published a study in which he had successfully isolated mycoplasma bacterium from the joints of rheumatic patients.[2] Mycoplasma is a very difficult bacterium to isolate and grow. In fact, it took Dr. Brown over three months and hundreds of experiments before he was able to isolate the bacterium. Other researchers (e.g., Williams[3] and Schaevorbeke, et al[4]) have also isolated mycoplasma in the joints of rheumatoid patients.

After isolating the bacteria in the joints of rheumatoid patients, Dr. Brown, former chairman of the Arthritis Institute in Virginia, embarked on a forty-year career of successfully using small doses of antibiotics to treat different arthritic conditions, including rheumatoid arthritis. This model of an infectious cause of some types of arthritis has been verified in animal studies as well and will be discussed further in the Discussion section.

With the advent of more sophisticated testing (i.e., Polymerase Chain Reaction, or PCR), the theory that mycoplasma may be the causative factor in some forms of arthritis has been further advanced. In 1999, with the use of PCR, Aristo Vojdani, Ph.D, found elevated levels of mycoplasma in the serum of patients suffering from rheumatoid arthritis, fibromyalgia, chronic fatigue syndrome and Gulf War Syndrome.[5]

Based upon my clinical experience, I agree with Dr. Brown's conclusion that many forms of arthritis have an infectious etiology and that patients will respond positively (often dramatically) to antibiotic therapy.

Case Studies

Carol is a 37-year-old corporate president. She was diagnosed with juvenile rheumatoid arthritis at two years of age. At that time, Carol had various symptoms of arthritis including pain in her knees and ankles. At the age of 28, Carol had breast augmentation, and she felt her body deteriorate after the surgery. "I felt like I was dying," she said. Carol had the implants removed a short time later, but the arthritic condition continued to worsen. Before Carol had reached the age of 31, both of her hips had been replaced. Her arthritic condition continued to worsen over the next few years. When I first saw Carol, her muscles and joints were incredibly stiff and painful and she had to walk with the assistance of a cane. Test results showed that she had very high antibody levels to mycoplasma bacterium as well as many nutritional and hormonal deficiencies. "I was stunned. How could someone discover so many new things about me when I had seen so many doctors?" Carol asked. I treated Carol with IV antibiotics and oral antibiotics. In addition, I prescribed natural hormones (Armour Thyroid, natural testosterone and natural progesterone) and a nutritional program, including vitamins (Vitamin C, Vitamin E, Vitamin D and Vitamin B12), minerals (zinc and copper), and herbs (Cats Claw, Licorice Root and others). Carol said, "Before starting the program, I could not freely shop or function; now I can walk anywhere. I can move and I am much more flexible. I experience far less pain and I am extremely energetic. Prior to the program, I could barely awaken in the morning and was always cold and tired. I am much stronger and I feel healthier than I have felt in my entire adult life. To understand that my immune system had been compromised from the time I incurred the bacteria, that it continued to be severely compromised by my breast implantation, and that these factors virtually led to the further destruction of my body's regulatory systems, is so logical to me. It is simply profound." Carol made these tremendous gains in her health in only eight months. In fact, she noticed an improvement in her condition within one month after starting the antibiotic therapy. Carol's physical therapist called me shortly after Carol had started the antibiotics to ask me what I was prescribing for her. The physical therapist was seeing great changes in the tone and function of Carol's muscles. "I have been working with Carol for five years and I have never seen such a dramatic improvement in her condition in such a short time," the physical therapist said.

Many times those with arthritis will find that their arthritic symptoms flare up after a surgery. If one has an infectious process (i.e., mycoplasma), surgery can trigger acceleration of the infectious process. Furthermore, silicone breast implants may accelerate immune system disorders such as arthritis.

In treating many different forms of arthritis, I have found that the antibiotic therapy is more effective when it is combined with the use of vitamins, minerals, herbs and natural hormones to improve the functioning of the immune system. Perhaps these arthritic individuals are more susceptible to infectious agents and are more prone to chronic disease because their bodies are lacking these basic nutrients.

Andy, age 18, had suffered from rheumatoid arthritis for four years. He was healthy until the age of 14 when he began to have pain in his knee. The pain became progressively worse and he was diagnosed with rheumatoid arthritis one year later. By then, he had pain in both knees and in his hands. "I used to be able to play sports; now it hurts too much," Andy lamented. He was treated with anti-inflammatory medications, including steroids. Andy said, "I couldn't stand how I felt. My stomach hurt and I became very angry on the medications." Andy's regimen was changed to gold injections with little success. He developed tremendous side effects, including fatigue and canker sores, from the gold injections. When Andy first came to me as a patient, I tested him for mycoplasma. Andy had high antibody levels in his blood, indicating a chronic infection with mycoplasma. In addition, he was found to have low levels of zinc, essential fatty acids and B vitamins. I treated Andy with Minocin (an antibiotic effective for treating mycoplasma bacteria), flaxseed oil, zinc, Vitamin B6, and Vitamin B complex 100. Within one month of this therapy, Andy noticed a marked improvement. "I feel 75% better. I no longer wake up stiff and I feel like I am getting my mobility back. This is the first time since I have been sick that I finally feel like I am getting better," he claimed.

Andy has now been treated with this regimen for over one year, and he continues to make steady progress. He is active in sports, suffers almost no pain and swelling in his joints, and now has a normal life. In addition, he has no side effects from the antibiotics.

By the age of 61, Judy had suffered with psoriatic arthritis for fifteen years. She had constant pain in her hands and knees, and her left knee was always swollen. "Sometimes I have difficulty walking up a flight of stairs," she said. She was unable to do her laundry because she could not carry the laundry down to the basement. Judy had seen a rheumatologist who wanted to put her on chemotherapeutic drugs. She refused. She stated, "Why should I take drugs that only treat the symptoms and don't treat the cause of the illness? Furthermore, when I learned about the side effects of these drugs, I decided there had to be a better way." Judy did the research on her own. On the Internet she found information about antibiotic therapy from the Road Back Foundation (a non-profit group designed to promote Dr. Brown's work with antibiotic treatments). Judy approached her rheumatologist about using antibiotic treatments and the rheumatologist begrudgingly put her on oral Minocin (antibiotic). Judy reported to the doctor that she felt better with the antibiotic but she would like to try the intravenous (IV) antibiotic therapy promoted by the Road Back Foundation. (See Discussion section.) The rheumatologist refused. "He wanted to take me off of the antibiotic, even though I was feeling better, and put me on a toxic drug. Not a chance," she stated. When I started treating Judy with a course of IV antibiotics (IV Doxycycline), she immediately improved. "Right after the first IV was going in me, I felt the swelling in my knees go down," Judy said. Judy has been receiving IV treatments every month for three years and her condition continues to improve. She can now walk up and down the stairs without difficulty. The constant swelling that she used to have in her knees is almost gone. Judy was found to be allergic to gluten (a common allergy with arthritics); and when she removed gluten from her diet, she had further improvement in her condition. I also treated Judy with the adrenal hormone DHEA. (See Chapter 5.) In addition, she was found to have elevated mercury levels in her body, probably due to her dental (amalgam) fillings. Upon removal of her fillings and undergoing an appropriate detoxification program (i.e., taking the oral chelating agent DMSA--covered in Chapter 10), coupled with vitamin and mineral supplementation, Judy's health continued to improve. (For more information on nutritional supplementation and detoxification, see Chapters 9 and 10.)

The cause of psoriatic arthritis is unknown. In conventional medicine there is usually little thought given to an infectious etiology. Without knowing (or even searching for) a cause, how can an effective treatment be prescribed? The conventional treatment of psoriatic arthritis often includes the use of nonsteroidal anti-inflammatory drugs (i.e., NSAID's).[6] Studies have shown that the prolonged use of these agents will actually inhibit healing in the injured joints.[7] If NSAID's fail, often toxic chemotherapy drugs are employed. I believe it is much safer and wiser to start with an appropriate antibiotic therapy when it is indicated. I have found patients with psoriatic arthritis respond very well to antibiotic therapy and have an improved response when it is combined with a proper nutritional evaluation and detoxification of the body.

Rene, age 57, was diagnosed with vasculitis four years ago. Vasculitis is an inflammatory disease of unknown origin that causes pain and inflammation throughout the body, particularly in the legs. The conventional treatment for vasculitis involves the use of chemotherapeutic agents designed to suppress the immune system. Rene tried to take cyclophosphamide (a chemotherapeutic agent) but could not tolerate the side effects. "The drug was worse than the illness," she said. "It gave me terrible headaches and made me exhausted." Rene also developed severe pain in her joints and was developing arthritic symptoms all over her body. "I felt as if I were aging incredibly fast. My doctors could not tell me what was causing this. They kept saying it was my immune system attacking my body. When I asked them why my own immune system would attack my body, they could not answer the question." When I first saw Rene, I found her to have a mycoplasma infection. She was immediately started on intravenous antibiotics (Clindamycin- 900mg twice per day for five days). She noticed an immediate improvement in her symptoms. "The rash that I had on my legs began to go away after the third IV was given to me. Also, the pain began to decrease. By the end of the IV's, I had almost no pain." After the IV treatments were completed, Rene was placed on the antibiotic Minocin. " It was a miracle. I began to feel much better," she exclaimed. Rene was further treated with natural hormones (DHEA, natural testosterone and natural hydrocortisone), as well as a vitamin and mineral regimen (Vitamin B6, magnesium and pycnogenols). It has been two years since Rene began the treatment, and she now feels that her condition is 80% improved. "I feel as if I have awakened from a bad dream. When I have pain episodes now, I can deal with them. I have been given my life back," she happily reports.

Vasculitis is classified as an autoimmune disorder. I have found that a high percentage of patients with vasculitis (as well as many other autoimmune disorders) often respond favorably to antibiotic therapy. Autoimmune disorders can be further improved with the addition of natural hormones, vitamins, minerals and herbs.

Discussion

Many arthritic diseases are classified as "autoimmune" diseases. An autoimmune disorder refers to a condition whereby the immune system produces antibodies against its own tissue, thus causing inflammation and destruction. In other words, the body is literally destroying its own tissue. Some examples of autoimmune arthritic disorders include rheumatoid arthritis, vasculitis, psoriatic arthritis and Lupus.

Perhaps many of the illnesses classified as autoimmune are not truly autoimmune disorders. One theory, known as "molecular mimicry," states that parts of an infectious bacterium may resemble structures of the body. For example, in many cases of arthritis, certain structures of the bacterial organism may resemble the tissue lining the joints of the body. As the body tries to mount an antibody response against the organism, these antibodies inadvertently attack the tissue lining of the joints resulting in joint destruction and inflammation. The correct treatment regimen in this case would be directed at destroying the organism. This is where antibiotic therapies hold promise in treating diseases like rheumatoid arthritis, psoriatic arthritis, Lupus, scleroderma and others. (See Table 1 for other diseases that may have an infectious etiology.)

Pharmacologic treatments directed only at inflammation in the body will not provide a long-term benefit or cure for such autoimmune diseases. Furthermore, the continued use of these medications may allow an infection to continue unabated in the body, thereby producing more destruction. Conventional treatments like NSAID's and other drug therapies have failed because these treatments focus solely on the inflammation (i.e., the symptom) instead of treating the infection (i.e., the cause). In other words, drug therapies do not treat the cause of any illness;

they only address the symptoms of disease. I believe that there is a bacterial origin for many disorders labeled as "autoimmune" and that unless the underlying cause (i.e., the infectious process) is properly treated, the illness will not improve.

The Arthritis-Infection Connection in Animals

It has been known for over one hundred years that mycoplasma organisms are able to cause arthritis symptoms in animals. In 1898, investigators isolated a strain of mycoplasma from cattle, and it was shown to cause arthritis in these cattle. Similar arthritis-producing organisms have been isolated from other animals, including cats, dogs, pigs, goats, sheep, turkeys, rats, mice, and gorillas.

Medical researchers search for clues of diseases in humans by trying to duplicate the illness and validate the treatment in an animal model. For over one hundred years there have been reports of isolating mycoplasma from animals who have arthritis and reports of inducing arthritis with exposure to and infection by mycoplasma. In fact, the arthritis in these animals and the arthritis in humans have very similar characteristics. There have also been numerous reports of arthritic animals whose symptoms have improved with the use of antibiotics.

The most celebrated report of an animal with arthritis was Tomoka, a gorilla at the National Zoo. Tomoka developed a case of rheumatoid arthritis at the age of five. He exhibited signs of extreme pain and would spend his time sitting in a corner rubbing his joints. Over twenty different arthritic treatments used in humans had failed with Tomoka. He failed to grow and there were plans to euthanize him. After all the options were exhausted, Dr. Brown was called in to evaluate Tomoka. Dr. Brown commented, "It soon became clear that we were seeing the first model of human rheumatoid arthritis ever encountered in an animal."[8]

Dr. Brown treated Tomoka with IV tetracycline (the same treatment he was giving to his human patients). Tomoka gradually improved, gaining full weight and strength. Within three years of receiving treatments, Tomoka resumed a normal, healthy life. Through twenty years of follow-up, there was no recurrence of his disease. Since the treatment of Tomoka, gorillas around the country have been treated in a similar fashion with remarkable results.

Garth Nicolson, M.D., found evidence of mycoplasma infection in a variety of chronic illnesses, including fibromyalgia, chronic fatigue syndrome and Gulf War Syndrome.[9] As mentioned before, Dr. Vojdani also found evidence of a bacterial infection in patients with chronic fatigue syndrome, fibromyalgia, rheumatoid arthritis and Gulf War Syndrome.[10] I have found particular success in using antibiotics (when indicated) in patients suffering from chronic fatigue syndrome and fibromyalgia.

Kim, a 38-year-old pharmaceutical sales representive, has suffered with fibromyalgia for over six years. Kim was well until she got the flu six years ago. " I never felt like I recovered from that flu," Kim said. " I used to feel pretty good, and I used to work out all of the time. I don't understand what has happened to me. My muscles always ache, and I have headaches all of the time. I feel like I have aged forty years since I became ill." Kim was taking NSAIDS and sleeping pills to help her sleep at night. "The medication does help somewhat, but I still feel lousy. I want to have children, but I don't feel strong enough to go through with a pregnancy," she said. Kim also exhibited signs of a hormonal imbalance: irregular and painful menstrual periods, fatigue, cold hands and feet, dry skin and hair loss. Kim's basal body temperature was very low at 96.4 degrees Fahrenheit. The normal temperature is 97.8-98.2 degrees Fahrenheit. I diagnosed Kim with hypothyroidism (see Chapter 4) and a mycoplasma infection. Kim was treated for hypothyroidism with natural thyroid hormone and for the mycoplasma infection with Minocin (oral antibiotic) three days per week. In addition, she was treated with vitamins (Vitamin B6-250mg/day, B-Complex- 1/day, Vitamin C-5000 mg/day), minerals (Magnesium- 400mg/day and Selenium-400mcg/day) and herbs (Cats Claw-1000mg/day). Her improvement was dramatic; within seven days she began to feel better. "It was a miracle. I began to feel better right away. The aching in my muscles immediately began to subside. I began to get my energy level back and started exercising again. I haven't been able to exercise at all for the past six years because it fatigued me too much," she said. Now, two years later, Kim feels 95% better. She claims, "I feel like I have my life back and I feel like I can do anything."

I have found that many patients with fibromyalgia (and chronic fatigue syndrome) often have concomitant bacterial infections. My experience has shown that these individuals will not achieve the best results unless the infectious process is properly diagnosed and treated. The best results are often achieved when the patient is treated holistically. The most effective treatment uses multiple therapies that treat the underlying cause of an illness and build up the body's immune system. This can include the use of vitamins, minerals and herbs along with antibiotics (when indicated). I have found that using a combination of therapies is much more effective than using individual therapies.

At the age of 17, Sandy's life was miserable. She was diagnosed with fibromyalgia when she was 15 years old. Sandy also suffered from migraine headaches as often as three days per week. Sandy's mother had to pull her out of school because she was having such a difficult time concentrating. "I feel miserable most of the time. My muscles ache and I always have some form of a headache. I used to love gymnastics; now there is no way I can do any sports. I am in too much pain and I am too tired," Sandy said. In addition, her menstrual periods had become very painful; and she had a large amount of bleeding with her periods. Sandy's physician treated her with NSAIDS and antidepressants. "I couldn't take the medication," she said. " The medication gave me stomach aches and made my brain foggy. Throughout this entire time period, Sandy exhibited many of the signs of hypothyroidism: cold hands and feet, dry skin, hair falling out, weight gain and constipation. (See Chapter 4.) Her basal body temperature averaged 96.6 degrees Fahrenheit. The normal temperature is 97.8-98.2 degrees Fahrenheit. I diagnosed Sandy's problem as a mycoplasma infection and hypothyroidism. Sandy began taking natural thyroid hormone and Minocin three days per week, and her condition dramatically improved. "Within one week of starting the medications, all of my problems began to improve. My muscles stopped aching, I was not cold any more and my periods became much easier. I felt as if a cloud was lifted off me," she said. Sandy was able to return to school as well as gymnastics six months after starting the medication. "I feel like a completely new person," Sandy says.

My experience has shown that many of those suffering from chronic illness such as fibromyalgia, will often have hormonal imbalances, particularly thyroid imbalances. Fibromyalgia is further discussed in Chapter 3. In addition, many of these patients can have concomitant bacterial infections, such as mycoplasma. Often, the best results are seen when combination therapies are used. In Sandy's case, she was treated with a combination of natural thyroid hormone and antibiotics. Natural hormones are further discussed in Chapters 4 and 5.

Anna, age 38, was diagnosed by her rheumatologist with

rheumatoid arthritis after the birth of her daughter three years ago. She developed acute onset of joint pain and swelling two months after her daughter was born. "Within two months of delivering my baby, I became extremely ill. I went to the best doctors and asked them why I was suddenly ill, since I had been feeling so good before. The only thing they could say was that I had an autoimmune disease," Anna said. "They could not explain to me why my body was attacking itself. I was in so much pain I didn't think I would be able to care for my baby." Anna was also diagnosed with Hashimoto's disease (an autoimmune condition of the thyroid gland). She was treated with steroids and NSAIDS for the pain and Levothyroxine (Levothroid) for the thyroid problem. When I saw Anna for the first time, she appeared older than her age. She also had swelling in her joints and puffiness of her face, and she was very fatigued and complained of being in pain most of the time. Anna commented that she did not want to have more children because she didn't think she could adequately care for another child in her condition. When I diagnosed Anna with a mycoplasma infection (Mycoplasma Hominis), she was ecstatic. "I hope this is why I am sick. The other doctors could not provide me with a rational reason of why I became so ill. This makes sense to me," she said. I treated Anna with IV Clindamyacin (see IV Antibiotic Section below) and oral Minocin. Within one month of starting the antibiotic therapy, Anna's condition dramatically improved. "I could not believe the difference. The swelling and the pain began to improve within one week. I feel like I used to feel, which is wonderful," she stated. I changed Anna's thyroid medication to natural thyroid hormone, Armour Thyroid (see Chapter 4). After evaluating a hair analysis, I also treated her condition with vitamins (Vitamin C, Vitamin E and Coenzyme Q-10) and minerals (copper, zinc, sea salt and magnesium). Anna's symptoms completely disappeared after being on this program for six months. "I feel so well now," she commented, "that my husband and I have decided to have more children. I could not have tolerated more children the way I was feeling before."

I have found wonderful results with treating many rheumatoid arthritic patients with the antibiotic therapy. As in Anna's case, the best results are often achieved by combining different therapies, (such as antibiotics with natural hormones, vitamins, minerals and herbs), rather than using a single modality. Many times, patients with arthritic disorders such as rheumatoid arthritis are so depleted nutritionally that they need proper nutritional support along with any other therapy provided. In Anna's case, she received the optimum result by adding natural items to her antibiotic regimen.

Trials Supporting the Use of Antibiotics to Treat Arthritis

A study at the University of London showed that the use of Minocin in severe rheumatoid arthritic patients improved most of the clinical variables measured, including pain and joint mobility.[11] The positive results with Minocin were further seen in studies in Israel[12] and the Netherlands.[13]

At the University of Nebraska, researchers looked at the response of patients recently diagnosed with early rheumatoid arthritis. Results showed a significant response in those who took Minocycline versus a placebo.[14] The largest study to date, known as the MIRA trial (Minocycline Treatment in Rheumatoid Arthritis), also showed a favorable improvement with those who took Minocycline.[15]

When I have used antibiotics to treat many of the conditions listed in Table 1, my experience has been very positive. I believe that many of these chronic illnesses may have an infectious cause. This infectious etiology is often ignored in conventional medicine. If the infectious cause is not properly treated, it will be nearly impossible to overcome the illnesses listed in Table 1. My clinical experience has shown that with the appropriate use of antibiotics, patients can recover from many of these chronic conditions.

Herxheimer Reactions

Occasionally after starting the antibiotic therapy, a worsening of symptoms occurs. This reaction is known as the

Herxheimer reaction and reflects the destruction of the organism (e.g., mycoplasma) and the body's difficulty with the removal of the organism. I have found wonderful results using holistic modalities, including IV nutritional therapies and oral vitamins and minerals, to ameliorate the Herxheimer affect. Also, drinking adequate amounts of water (see Chapter 8) helps reduce the Herxheimer reaction. Digestive enzymes are another wonderful aid in blocking the Herxheimer reaction.

Intravenous Antibiotics Are Also Helpful

Dr. Brown found that combining a short course of intravenous (IV) antibiotics with the oral treatments (e.g., Minocin) provided a better response than using the oral antibiotics alone. Similarly, I have found better results with using a short course (usually five days) of IV antibiotics for treating patients with arthritis.

In my experience with arthritic patients, the best results have been achieved by administering a five-day course of IV antibiotics (usually Clindamyacin) before starting the oral antibiotics. IV antibiotics are helpful for treating those suffering with a mycoplasma infection for the following reasons:

1. Mycoplasma bacteria can colonize deeply in the tissue, and IV antibiotics can reach more deeply into the tissue than oral antibiotics.

2. IV antibiotics can bypass the gastrointestinal system and, therefore, can be more concentrated than the oral medications.

3. Most individuals with a chronic illness such as arthritis have a depressed immune system (sometimes compounded by having used drugs that further suppress the immune system); and they are more susceptible to infection by a variety of organisms, including mycoplasma. IV antibiotics are much more likely to cover a broad range of organisms than the sole use of oral antibiotics.

I have found that IV antibiotics can be a wonderful adjunctive treatment to the oral antibiotic treatment outlined in this chapter. When I started using antibiotics to treat chronic conditions such as arthritis, I immediately observed positive results in my patients. After combining IV antibiotic therapy with the oral antibiotic therapy, I observed a much better response. At a recent conference of the Road Back Foundation, the use of IV antibiotics was validated by the physicians who employ it in their practice in the treatment of many different arthritic illnesses.

Patti, age 41, began suffering from a mild case of chronic fatigue at age 26. Approximately one year later, she started developing joint pain. She said, "I got up for work and my thumb was very sore. I thought I just slept on it wrong. This went away after a few weeks, but then my arm started hurting. The arm would stop hurting after a few days, and then a different joint would start hurting. After the birth of my son eight years ago, things worsened. The pain and fatigue intensified. My hands were so swollen, I had difficulty changing my son's diapers." Patti went to a rheumatologist who diagnosed her with rheumatoid arthritis. "The doctor told me to do everything I want to do now because this autoimmune disease is only going to get worse. He told me to take Tylenol for pain; and when that stopped working, he had four immune suppressants to offer me. I left in tears. A few days later, I got mad and started reading. One night I heard a doctor on the radio talking about using antibiotics to treat rheumatoid arthritis. I had to beg my doctor for the antibiotics. Two months after starting the oral antibiotic (Minocin), I began to feel better. When I added a second antibiotic (Zithromax, taken two days per week), I felt better than ever. The pain, swelling and fatigue were all improving," Patti commented. Then, about a year ago, Patti developed a Herxheimer reaction and found herself in a wheelchair. When I first saw Patti, she could barely walk. After evaluating her, I placed her on vitamins and minerals with IV vitamin therapies. I also started treatment with the IV antibiotic Clindamyacin, along with natural hormones: natural thyroid (Chapter 4), DHEA, natural progesterone and natural testosterone (Chapter 5). She quickly came out of the Herxheimer Reaction. "After starting the IV treatments, I finally felt like the fight was over. I quickly put the wheelchair away, as I no longer needed it," Patti said. After one year of this treatment, Patti only complained of pain in her knees. I recently gave Patti two injections of the antibiotic Clindamyacin in her knees. Within one month of the injections, the swelling and warmth in both knees began to subside. "I can't believe how much better I feel. My husband just bought me a tandem bike, and we have started bicycle riding. Can you believe it? Me bicycle riding with my family! The fatigue is totally gone, and I feel like I will continue to improve," Patti commented to me.

Patti's story is not unusual. Adding intravenous antibiotics to the oral antibiotics is often extremely helpful. The IV antibiotic treatments are synergistic with the oral treatments. In addition, I have observed success in injecting the joints of arthritic patients with Clindamyacin. Patients who are responding to oral antibiotics will usually have a favorable response to intravenous antibiotics. Finally, I have found, as in Patti's case, the addition of IV nutritional therapies to be a wonderful benefit to those who suffer from a chronic condition.

Why Has Such A Promising Treatment Been Overlooked?

If antibiotics are such a helpful treatment for many people who suffer from arthritis and other conditions, why hasn't this therapy become more widely accepted in conventional medicine? The answer to this question goes back fifty years.

In the early 1900's, most research in arthritis focused on an infectious etiology. Researchers knew that arthritis in animals was often caused by certain bacteria (i.e., mycoplasma). Researcher Albert Sabin found that when mice were injected with mycoplasma, they developed arthritis.[16] Dr. Thomas Brown was able to isolate mycoplasma from the joint of a rheumatoid arthritic patient. He immediately began treating patients with antibiotics (tetracycline or Minocin) that inhibit mycoplasma and found positive results.

In the late 1940's, just as Dr. Brown was reporting positive results treating arthritics with antibiotics, cortisone was discovered. Initial uses of cortisone had dramatic effects on patients. Dr. Brown writes, "It was absolutely astonishing to see its (cortisone's) effects on patients who had been bed-ridden with crippling, advanced rheumatoid arthritis: they were suddenly able to rise and walk again without pain."[17]

Medicine began to focus its energy and resources away from an infectious etiology of arthritis, and instead began to focus its resources on the theory that arthritics must produce smaller amounts of cortisone. Also, it was felt that there must be some "autoimmune" phenomenon of cortisol. However, this theory was flawed. Within a short time of using high doses of cortisol, adverse effects began appearing: cataracts, osteoporosis, diabetes, hypertension and others.

However, because of the initial improvement in very ill patients, most of the research from that time on, was devoted to finding drugs that abruptly relieved the symptoms of arthritis; forgoing the research into the infectious nature. Dr. Brown described the atmosphere in medicine at the time, "Nobody seemed to care what made arthritis happen as long as they could control the symptoms."[18]

As cortisone declined in popularity, pharmaceutical companies were quick to start producing nonsteroidal anti-inflammatory drugs. These drugs have the anti-inflammatory effects of cortisone but do not have many of the side effects.

Nonsteroidal anti-inflammatory drugs (NSAIDS) will initially provide relief of inflammation and pain in arthritic patients. However, as with cortisone, prolonged use of these drugs will result in serious side effects: bleeding, ulcers and others. Today, nearly forty years after the discovery of cortisone,

NSAID's are the standard of care in the initial treatment of arthritic patients. Yet, there is not a <u>single</u> study that shows NSAID's will cure or even reverse any form of arthritis. In fact, the opposite has been shown to be true: long-term use of NSAID's can actually worsen cases of arthritis. Dr. Brown theorizes that the inflammation around the joint (which the NSAID removes) is our body's way of trying to contain the infection. When the inflammation is removed without treating the cause, the infection, and therefore the disease process, is allowed to spread.

Pharmaceutical companies have made billions upon billions of dollars producing one NSAID after another. Doctors are given fascinating lectures about how the "newest" NSAID works better than the previous thirty versions. However, none of these products can claim to treat the cause of arthritis.

The other types of drugs used for arthritis, known as "Disease Modifying Anti-Rheumatic Drugs" (DMARD's) fare little better. Examples of these agents include gold injections, Methotrexate and steroids. These drugs are very toxic to the body, and close monitoring must follow the use of these drugs. Most of these drugs work by blocking inflammation in the body, but many other functions of them are unknown. These drugs are prone to very serious side effects, including kidney and liver damage.

One further explanation of why conventional medicine has failed to accept the infectious theory of diseases like arthritis is that the drugs (i.e., antibiotics) advocated by Dr. Brown, including Minocin and the tetracycline antibiotics, are beyond their patents.

When the pharmaceutical companies cannot hold an exclusive patent on a product, the profit margins are much lower. It is much more profitable for these companies to promote the use of patentable items, such as NSAIDS, versus non-patentable drugs like Minocin.

Medicine can be agonizingly slow to change. In the last five years, with the MIRA study and others, there is an increased interest in an infectious cause of certain forms of arthritis. I believe this interest will continue to grow. The antibiotic therapy is much safer and much less toxic than the other therapies mentioned. Furthermore, I see greater clinical efficacy in my patients with the proper use of antibiotics in the treatment of some forms of arthritis.

Antibiotics Are Not The Whole Story

Although I believe antibiotics should be considered in the treatment of many different forms of arthritis, I feel that antibiotics should not be the only treatment used in these illnesses.

Antibiotics are only effective when the immune system is optimally functioning. In order for the immune system to be optimally functioning, the body must have adequate amounts of vitamins and minerals. Also, the hormonal system must be properly balanced. Eating healthy food to nourish the immune system is a must. Finally, toxins must be removed from the body. All of these items are covered in much more depth in Chapters 3-11.

How To Diagnose a Mycoplasma Infection

There are many different ways to isolate a bacterium. The "gold standard" for diagnosing a bacterial infection is to culture (i.e., grow) the bacteria. Mycoplasma is a very difficult bacterium to isolate and grow in the body. Because it is so difficult to grow in a culture and because culturing of mycoplasma-infected tissue often turns up negative, many physicians and researchers doubt that mycoplasma bacterium is the cause of arthritis. However, the research does support the idea of mycoplasma as the cause of infections in man as well as in animals.

It is well known that mycoplasma can irreversibly bind to tissues in the body. This tight binding is what makes mycoplasma so difficult to culture. Dr. Harold Clark, a scientist who specialized in mycoplasma research, found that when mycoplasma was injected into animals (mice, rats and pigs), it produced arthritis. However, after producing arthritis, the mycoplasma could not be isolated from the animal. Dr. Clark reasoned this was the same binding mechanism used in humans.[19] Because the mycoplasma binds so tightly to the tissue, it is very difficult to grow in a culture. When the mycoplasma binds to the tissue (in arthritics the tissue is the joints), it produces an inflammatory response; and the signs and symptoms of arthritis appear.

If we cannot isolate the bacterium from the body, then how do we make the diagnosis? I have found that using antibody testing is the most reliable method to diagnose a mycoplasma infection. When there is an infection in the body, the body responds to the infection by producing substances called antibodies that bind to the bacteria (or virus) and help neutralize it.

Specific antibody testing can be done to see if the body is producing antibodies against mycoplasma infections. I have found The Arthritis Research Center in Bethesda, Maryland (phone number: 301-216-1231) to be the most reliable testing facility for the mycoplasma bacterium. This is the lab founded by Dr. Brown's laboratory director, Millicent Coker-Vann, Ph.D. This lab will check antibody levels for five different strains of mycoplasma. Also, Polymerase Chain Reaction (PCR) testing has proven to be very helpful in diagnosing a mycoplasma infection. Dr. Robert Franco, a rheumatologist in California who has successfully utilized antibiotic treatments for arthritis for over ten years, primarily uses PCR testing in his office. A good laboratory for PCR testing is Immunosciences Lab (phone number: 310-657-1077).

Proper testing should be done before instituting any therapy. Repeat testing should be done at intervals (six months to one year) to follow the progress. Mycoplasma testing should only be done at a laboratory experienced in working with the organism. Inexperienced labs can provide inaccurate results.

Final Thoughts

Whenever I place patients on antibiotic therapy, I recommend that they supplement with Lactobacillus Acidophilus. Lactobacillus Acidophilus is a bacterium that is normally present in a healthy gastrointestinal tract. Antibiotics can deplete Lactobacillus in the GI tract, resulting in an overgrowth of harmful bacteria and yeast. Supplementing with Lactobacillus Acidophilus helps to prevent this overgrowth and also helps to keep the immune system functioning at an optimal level.

There is no safer or more effective treatment than the judicious use of antibiotics in the treatment of many chronic illnesses. With appropriate evaluation and testing, this therapy should be offered to all patients who suffer from a chronic illness such as arthritis.

The Road Back Foundation is a non-profit organization that continues Dr. Brown's research on the treatment of arthritic disorders with antibiotics. For more information, you can contact the Road Back Foundation at the following address:

The Road Back Foundation
Box 447
Orleans, MA 02653
(508) 255-8422
www.roadback.org

[1] Clark, Harold. Why Arthritis? Searching for the cause and the Cure of Rheumatoid Disease. Axelrod Publishing. 1997

[2] Brown, Thomas. The Road Back. Evans Publishing. 1988

[3] Williams, M.H. "Pathogenic mycoplasma in rheumatoid arthritis?" Ciba Foundation Symposium. Amsterdam: Associated Scientific Publishers, 1972; 251-262

[4] Schaevorbeke, Thierry, et al. "Mycoplasma Fermentans in joints of patients with rheumatoid arthritis and other joint disorders." Lancet. Vol. 347. 5/18/96, p. 1418

[5] Vojdani, Aristo, et al. "Multiplex PCR for the Detection of Mycoplasma fermentans, M. hominis, and M. penetrans in Patients with Chronic Fatigue Syndrome, Fibromyalgia, Rheumatoid Arthritis and Gulf War Syndrome." Journal of Chronic Fatigue Syndrome. Vol. 5. No. 314, 1999 p. 187-197.

[6] Harrison's Principals of Internal Medicine, 14th edition, 1998. P. 1950.

[7] Rashad, S et al. "Effect of non-steroidal anti-inflammatory drugs on the course of osteoarthritis." Lancet. 1989;2:519-522

[8] Brown, Thomas. The Road Back. Evans Publishing. 1988.

[9] Nicolson, Garth et al. "Mycoplasmal Infections in chronic illnesses: Fibromyalgia and chronic fatigue syndromes, gulf war illness, HIV-Aids and rheumatoid arthritis." Medical Sentinel. Volume 4, Number 5. 1999

[10] Vojdani et al. IBID.

[11] Breedveld, FC, et al. "Minocycline treatment for rheumatoid arthritis: An open dose finding study." J. Rheumatology. 17:43, 1990

[12] Langevitz, P, et al. "Treatment of resistant arthritis with Minocycline: An open study." J. Rheumatology. 19: 1502, 1992

[13] Kloppenburg, M et al. "Antibiotics as disease modifiers in arthritis." Clin. Exp. Rheum. 9\8:s113, 1993

[14] Odell, James et al. "Treatment of early seropositive rheumatoid arthritis with Minocycline." Arthritis and Rheumatism. Vol. 42, No. 8, August 1999, p. 1691-95

[15] Tilley, BC et al. "Minocycline in rheumatoid arthritis: A 48-week double blind, placebo-controlled trial." Ann. Intern. Med 122:81, 1995

[16] Brown, Thomas. IBID, p. 222.

[17] Brown, Thomas. IBID p. 150

[18] Brown, Thomas. IBID. p. 152

[19] Clark, Harold. IBID. p. 49

Chapter 3

Fibromyalgia and Chronic Fatigue Syndrome

Related Conditions: Fibromyalgia and Chronic Fatigue Syndrome

I have found that many different illnesses will respond to the holistic approaches I have outlined in this book. This chapter will focus on two conditions: fibromyalgia and chronic fatigue syndrome. Though the primary focus of this book is on the holistic treatments for arthritis, I felt it would be incomplete if it did not adequately address these two related conditions.

Fibromyalgia is a chronic disorder characterized by poor sleep, muscle pain, stiffness and tender trigger points on the body. Fibromyalgia and chronic fatigue syndrome share many of the same symptoms. A diagnosis of fibromyalgia does not exclude a second clinical diagnosis, such as chronic fatigue syndrome or arthritis. I find that many of my patients who have one chronic disorder (e.g., arthritis) often have many of the signs and symptoms to meet the criteria for a diagnosis of fibromyalgia. The criteria for the diagnosis of fibromyalgia from the American College of Rheumatology are given on the next page.

ACR Definition of Fibromyalgia Syndrome

1. A history of widespread pain for at least three months. Pain is considered widespread when all of the following are present: pain in the left side of the body, the right side of the body, below the waist and above the waist. In addition, there should be axial pain (cervical spine or anterior chest or thoracic spine or low back).
2. Pain in trigger points on the neck, back, hips, arms and legs.

Revised CDC Criteria for Chronic Fatigue Syndrome. A case of chronic fatigue syndrome is defined by the presence of the following:

1. Clinically evaluated, unexplained, persistent or relapsing fatigue that is of new or definite onset; is not the result of ongoing exertion; is not alleviated by rest; and results in substantial reduction of previous levels of occupational, educational, social or personal activities.
2. Four or more of the following symptoms that persist or recur during six or more consecutive months of illness and that do not predate the fatigue:
   a. Self-reported impairment in short-term memory or concentration
   b. Sore throat
   c. Tender cervical or axillary nodes
   d. Muscle pain
   e. Multijoint pain without redness or swelling
   f. Headaches of a new pattern or severity
   g. Unrefreshing sleep
   h. Postexertional malaise lasting > 24 hours

Chronic fatigue syndrome also shares many of the same characteristics with fibromyalgia. These characteristics include unexplained fatigue, poor sleep, muscle pain, poor memory, headaches and others.[1] Often it is difficult to clinically distinguish between the two disorders. The diagnostic criteria for fibromyalgia and chronic fatigue syndrome are listed on the previous page.

The incidence of fibromyalgia and chronic fatigue syndrome is staggering. It is estimated that between three and six million people in the United States currently suffer from chronic fatigue and/or fibromyalgia.

The cause of chronic fatigue syndrome and fibromyalgia is unknown. There are many theories as to why these illnesses develop, including the following: infections (viral, bacterial, fungal and parasitic), hormonal disturbances, toxicity, nutritional deficiencies, immune disturbances, allergies (food and environmental) and others. Often patients with chronic fatigue syndrome and fibromyalgia will have many of the above problems coexisting at the same time.

Researchers have shown a link between mycoplasma infections and fibromyalgia and chronic fatigue syndrome. Aristo Vojdani, Ph.D., found 54% of individuals with fibromyalgia and 52% of individuals with chronic fatigue syndrome had evidence of a mycoplasma infection. Only 15% of healthy individuals had signs of a mycoplasma infection.[2] Another researcher, Garth Nicolson, Ph.D., found that 70% of individuals suffering from fibromyalgia or chronic fatigue syndrome tested positive for a mycoplasma infection. In this study, only 9% of healthy individuals were found to have evidence of a mycoplasma infection.[3]

There is not one causative factor for fibromyalgia or chronic fatigue. The causative factor (or factors) can vary from one individual to the next. In other words, one patient with fibromyalgia may be suffering from a viral illness while another with the same diagnosis may have a nutritional deficiency. As mentioned before, almost all who suffer from these illnesses will have numerous causative factors occurring at the same time. It is imperative to simultaneously evaluate all possible causative factors (outlined above) and to treat all of these factors concurrently.

My experience has shown that it is not effective to use a single treatment modality to treat these chronic conditions. In these illnesses, one condition can trigger other conditions (e.g., a viral illness can trigger a hormonal imbalance). A single treatment modality will not achieve the optimum results in these patients.

Because patients with fibromyalgia and chronic fatigue syndrome have multiple problems occurring simultaneously, only a holistic approach will be effective. My experience has shown that all of the different treatment options outlined in this book (e.g., antibiotic therapy, natural hormonal therapies, nutritional therapies, detoxification and others) need to be appropriately assessed and used in order to achieve an optimum outcome. In addition, using these therapies in combination with one another is much more effective than using the therapies individually. Conventional medicine's reliance on using one drug to treat an illness is not effective in these chronic conditions.

Case Studies

Michelle, age 39, suffered with fibromyalgia for seven years. "I became ill with the flu seven years ago, and I feel like I have never recovered. I ache all over and never feel rested. I feel like an old lady," she lamented. When I examined Michelle, I found her to have numerous hormonal imbalances, including a hypothyroid condition and a hypoadrenal condition. Her basal body temperatures averaged 96.6 degrees Fahrenheit (normal is 97.8-98.2 degrees Fahrenheit), and her DHEA level was 390ng/ml (normal for women is 1,500-2,500ng/dl). Also, a 24-hour urine analysis showed Michelle was very low on hydrocortisone. (Her 17-OH steroid level was 3.0 mg/24 hours; normal is 7-10mg/24 hours.) After Michelle began treatment with natural thyroid hormone and the adrenal hormones DHEA and hydrocortisone, she noticed an immediate improvement. "Within one week of starting the hormones, I began to feel like I was waking up from a deep sleep. My head became clearer, and my aching began to diminish. It was a miracle. I couldn't remember when I had felt this good," she said. Michelle was further treated with vitamins (Vitamin A, Vitamin E and Vitamin D) and minerals (selenium, magnesium, iodine and others) and herbs (gingko biloba, silymarin and others). Today, nearly three years later, Michelle feels that her fibromyalgia symptoms have improved by 90%.

Fibromyalgia is a very difficult condition to treat. There is no known cause of fibromyalgia, and currently there is no effective treatment in conventional medicine. There may not be one single cause of fibromyalgia; but people with this illness will share many of the same signs and symptoms, including hormonal imbalances.

I have found that thyroid and adrenal imbalances exist in most patients who suffer from fibromyalgia. Also, the majority of patients suffering from this illness have severe nutritional deficiencies. Furthermore, many of my patients have heavy metal toxicities. (Heavy metal toxicities are covered in more detail in Chapter 10.) Until these imbalances and toxicities are properly diagnosed and treated, there will often be a sub-optimal response to any therapy.

At age 35, Sherri was miserable from fibromyalgia. "I can't sleep at night. I am awake all night looking at the alarm clock. My husband can't sleep in the same bed with me because I toss and turn all night," she said. Sherri was diagnosed with fibromyalgia approximately four years before I saw her. "After the birth of my third child, I could not recover," she claimed. "At first I thought it was because I was tired from taking care of the kids. After a while, I realized that something was wrong. However, when I went to the doctor, he kept telling me I was depressed." Sherri also complained of a twenty-pound weight gain that she could not lose. "I could stop eating and I still would not lose weight," she said. Furthermore, Sherri was always cold, complaining of constantly having cold hands and feet. "In the winter, I can't walk outside without gloves or my hands will turn purple and become extremely painful," she said. When I examined Sherri, I found she had many of the signs of hypothyroidism, including poor eyebrow growth, puffiness under the eyes and an enlarged tongue. Sherri's basal body temperature averaged 96.5 degrees Fahrenheit (normal is 97.8-98.2 degrees Fahrenheit). In addition, I found Sherri to have elevated antibody levels to the bacterium, mycoplasma. (See Chapter 2.) Sherri was appropriately placed on Armour Thyroid hormone, and she was treated with Minocycline (an antibiotic to treat mycoplasma) three days per week. In addition, she was given a short course of intravenous vitamin therapies to correct nutritional imbalances. Sherri began to feel better within one month. "After three or four weeks, I began to feel better. My energy began to come back, and I began to sleep better. The pain also began to subside," she said. Sherri has been treated with this regimen for two years, and she no longer has any symptoms of fibromyalgia. "I feel like I have been reborn. I no longer suffer from pain, and I can now play with my kids," she claims. Sherri's antibiotic therapy was stopped a short time after her blood tests showed that she no longer had mycoplasma in her blood. Today, Sherri remains in good health and continues to take vitamins (Vitamin C, Vitamin B6, Vitamin E), minerals (magnesium, selenium), herbs (Cat's Claw, Silymarin) and natural hormones (natural thyroid hormone) to support her *immune system.*

My experience has shown that many fibromyalgia patients have multiple problems occurring simultaneously, as was true in Sherri's case. Often times, these patients' immune systems are malfunctioning because of nutritional deficiencies, hormonal imbalances, infections, allergies (food and environmental) and other causes. Until all of these conditions are appropriately diagnosed and treated, these patients will have a very difficult time recovering from these illnesses. In Sherri's case, using an antibiotic, Minocin, was absolutely necessary to treat the mycoplasma infection. This was complemented with nutritional therapies and natural hormonal therapies. The immune system of patients suffering from fibromyalgia is often poorly functioning because of infectious agents and nutritional imbalances.

Phil, a 32-year-old engineer, had been diagnosed with chronic fatigue syndrome five years before I saw him. After seeking care from four doctors, he was told nothing could be done to help him. Though Phil was able to work, he had no life outside of work. "I used to enjoy sports; now I barely have the energy to watch sports on television. Also, I am cold all of the time, even when everyone else is complaining of how warm it is," Phil complained. Phil's basal temperature averaged 96.6 degrees, more than one degree below normal. He drank inordinately large amounts of caffeinated beverages in order to keep going, but to no avail. When Phil was started on Armour Thyroid hormone, he immediately noticed an improvement in his condition. Each time the dose was increased, he noticed further improvement. It took three months to finally achieve an adequate thyroid level (two grains), whereupon Phil felt as if he had "been reborn." Furthermore, his basal temperature improved to a healthy 98.0 degrees Fahrenheit. Phil was additionally treated with the adrenal hormone DHEA and nutritional supplements (Vitamin B6, Vitamin C, Vitamin B Complex, magnesium and others). Today, four years after starting these natural therapies, Phil remains symptom free. He is back to playing sports and claims, "I feel like I have the energy I had when I was in my twenties. I feel like a new person."

My experience has shown that a large percentage (more than seventy percent) of chronic fatigue patients are hypothyroid. Chronic fatigue syndrome is nearly impossible to overcome unless the hormonal system is appropriately evaluated and treated. Good health and a resolution of many conditions such as chronic fatigue syndrome is possible with the proper use of natural hormones and nutritional supplementation, as was illustrated in Phil's case.

Discussion

A diagnosis of fibromyalgia or chronic fatigue syndrome can be a devastating diagnosis. Conventional medicine has criteria for making the diagnosis of these illnesses, however there is no consensus on the causative factor(s) of these illnesses. In conventional circles, some of the proposed causes of these illnesses include viral infections (Epstein Barr Virus, Cytomegalovirus, Herpes Virus, etc), immune dysfunction and depression.

Conventional therapies for treating these diseases are almost non-existent. Conventional doctors frequently employ the use of nonsteroidal anti-inflammatory drugs and antidepressant drugs. These treatments only address the symptoms of the illness (inflammation and depression); they do not address the underlying causative factors. Treatments that only address the symptoms of an illness are bound to be ineffective. Furthermore, many drug therapies can be toxic to the body and actually worsen the illness. Natural remedies, on the other hand, are safer and more effective at treating chronic illnesses such as fibromyalgia and chronic fatigue syndrome.

As mentioned before, I believe the causes of these chronic conditions are multifaceted in nature. I have observed in my practice that nearly all of the patients with these illnesses exhibit many of the following conditions:

1. Hormonal dysfunction
2. Chronic infections (viral, bacterial or fungal)
3. Nutritional deficiencies
4. Heavy metal toxicities
5. Allergies (environmental and food)

The result of having the above conditions (either individually or in combination) is a poorly functioning immune system. Recent studies have found immune system dysfunction in those who suffer from these conditions.[4][5] I have seen very positive results in my practice by properly evaluating and treating all of the causative factors of chronic fatigue syndrome and fibromyalgia.

Hormonal Evaluation

When a patient comes into my office suffering from symptoms of fibromyalgia or chronic fatigue syndrome, I begin my evaluation by taking a history and doing a physical exam. I use the following blood tests to evaluate the hormonal system:

Thyroid: TSH, T3 total, T4 total

Adrenal: DHEA-Sulfate, Pregnenolone

Ovarian: Progesterone, Estradiol

Testicular: Testosterone total

Physiologic (i.e., small) doses of natural hormones can be used to correct deficient states of the above-mentioned hormones. A hormonal system in disarray will cause a poorly functioning immune system, which can result in the patient developing the signs and symptoms of fibromyalgia and chronic fatigue. I have found that using natural hormones to correct these imbalances can provide tremendous support to the immune system and can help relieve many of the symptoms of these illnesses. After beginning therapy, blood tests are monitored to ensure adequate absorption and utilization of these hormones. Further information on the use of natural hormones can be found in my book, The Miracle of Natural Hormones 2nd Edition.

Infections

When a patient exhibits the symptoms of fibromyalgia and chronic fatigue syndrome, I believe it is important to determine whether that patient is also suffering from a chronic infectious state. This can be accomplished with blood testing for antibody levels to different bacteria (e.g., mycoplasma—see Chapter 2) and viruses (e.g., Epstein-Barr Virus, Cytomegalovirus, etc.). Over time, a chronic infection will exhaust the immune system and can result in many of the symptoms of fibromyalgia and chronic fatigue syndrome (as well as those of many other disorders). Unless the infectious process is properly treated, it becomes difficult for the immune system to properly function and for patients to overcome their illness.

There are many research articles that support the hypothesis that an infection may be one cause of these illnesses.[6] [7] [8] Other chronic illnesses, including the autoimmune disorders (e.g., rheumatoid arthritis, scleroderma, Lupus, etc.), have also been related to an infectious etiology. It is unclear whether the infectious agent is the causative factor or an opportunistic infection that is responsible for aggravating patient morbidity.[9]   In either case, the infectious agent needs to be appropriately diagnosed and treated. (Further information on the infectious etiology of chronic illness can be found in Chapter 2.)

Nutritional Deficiencies

Nutritional deficiencies are very common in patients who suffer from fibromyalgia and chronic fatigue syndrome. It makes common sense that individuals suffering from a chronic illness need an appropriate nutritional evaluation to ensure that the body has the basic nutrients (i.e., vitamins, minerals and others) necessary for healing to take place. My experience has shown that individuals who suffer from these conditions often have multiple nutritional deficiencies.   These nutritional deficiencies must be addressed through the use of vitamins, minerals, herbs and other natural items.   Many researchers have also found nutrient deficiencies in these illnesses.[10] [11] [12] [13]

I test my patients for nutrient levels using serum (blood) tests, hair tests and urine tests. The most common deficiencies that I have observed include the following:

1.   B Vitamins (B12 and B6 are usually low in individuals with fibromyalgia and chronic fatigue)
2.   Vitamin D

3.   Magnesium
4.   Essential Fatty Acids (particularly Omega 3)
5.   Selenium

Though the above list does not contain all of the nutrients that can be deficient, these are the most common deficiencies I have observed.   Unless specific nutritional deficiencies are addressed, there will be a sub-optimal response to any therapy.

I recommend the following dosages of nutrients when levels are found to be sub-optimal:

1.   B   Complex   100:   2/day.   Vitamin   B12 (hydroxycobalamine form of B12 only) should be given via intramuscular injections: 1mg twice per week. B6: 200mg/day.

2.   Vitamin D: 1000-2000 IU/day.   Levels must be followed.

3.   Magnesium (chelated): 400-800mg/day

4.   Essential Fatty Acids (EFA's):   Levels should be checked.   An Omega 3 EFA deficiency, which is the most common type of EFA deficiency, requires supplementation with flax seed oil or EPA (fish oil). It is essential to use a reputable company. (See Chapter 9 for more information.)

5.   Selenium: 200-400mcg/day

Nutritional supplementation is only one part of the treatment plan to improve the health of those suffering from a chronic illness. For the best results the nutritional recommendations should be coupled with dietary strategies emphasizing foods containing high levels of these nutrients. (Further information on nutritional supplementation can be found in Chapter 9.)

Heavy Metal Toxicity

Heavy metal toxicity is another possibility that should be considered when diagnosing and treating fibromyalgia and chronic fatigue syndrome. Heavy metal toxicity wreaks havoc with one's immune system. Heavy metals include:

1. Lead
2. Mercury
3. Arsenic
4. Nickel
5. Cadmium

Heavy metals are toxins that can come from numerous sources, including industrial pollutants (in the air, water and soil) and dental fillings.

It is imperative for every patient with fibromyalgia, chronic fatigue syndrome, or any other chronic illness to be screened for heavy metal toxicity. Screening for toxicity can be performed with a hair analysis and a urine challenge test. (For further information on heavy metals and heavy metal testing, I refer the reader to Chapter 10.)

Allergies

When the immune system is not working properly, an individual is more likely to develop allergies. An allergy can be defined as a hypersensitive response by the immune system to an antigen. Many substances can be antigens: food, drugs, environmental substances (dust, mold, grass, etc.) and others. Often the more ill individuals become from illnesses such as fibromyalgia or chronic fatigue syndrome, the more allergic they will also become. Conversely, the symptoms of these illnesses subside when the allergic symptoms improve.

I believe all patients suffering from chronic fatigue syndrome and fibromyalgia should be screened for allergies. Removing offending allergens and treating the allergy symptoms can allow the immune system to function better. I have found an electro-dermal system (where a computer can check the body for allergic sensitivities) to be extremely helpful in screening for food and environmental allergies. Treating allergies with an acupressure technique known as NAET has been helpful in reversing many of my patients' allergies. (Further information on allergies and NAET can be found in Chapter 7.)

Final Thoughts

Treating a chronic illness such as fibromyalgia or chronic fatigue syndrome can be a daunting task. Conventional medicine has failed in the treatment of many chronic disorders. Drug therapies are generally unsuccessful because they usually treat the symptoms of the disease, not the underlying cause(s). Until the underlying cause is treated, full recovery is unlikely. In addition, drug therapies are often toxic to the body and can inhibit healing reactions in the body. However, by using a holistic treatment plan, it is possible to regain good health. The techniques I have outlined in this chapter and in this book have proven to be successful for hundreds of my patients. I strongly encourage the reader to explore holistic treatment options to help overcome illness and promote optimum health.

[1] Harrison's Principles of Internal Medicine, 14th Edition. McGraw Hill. 1998, p. 2484

[2] Vojdani, Aristo, et al. "Multiplex PCR for the Detection of Mycoplasma fermentans, M. Hominis, and M. Penetrans in Patients with Chronic Fatigue Syndrome, Fibromyalgia, Rheumatoid Arthritis, and Gulf War Syndrome." Journal of Chronic Fatigue Syndrome, Vol. 5., No ¾ 1999.

[3] Nicolson, Garth et al. Mycoplasma Infections in Chronic Illnesses: Fibromyalgia and Chronic Fatigue Syndromes, Gulf War Illness, HIV-AIDS and Rheumatoid Arthritis. Medical Sentinel. Volume 4, No. 5, September/October 1999.

[4] Bennett, A. L., et al. "Elevation of Bioactive Transforming Growth Factor-B in Serum from Patients with Chronic Fatigue Syndrome." Journal of Clinical Immunology 17. 1997. p. 160.

[5] Vojdani, A., et al. "Elevated apoptotic cell population in patients with chronic fatigue syndrome: the pivotal role of protein kinase RNA." Journal of Internal Medicine 242. 1997. p. 465

[6] Choppa, P.C., et al. "Multiplex PCR for the detection of Mycoplasma fermentans, M. hominis and M. Penetrans in cell cultures and blood samples of patients with chronic fatigue syndrome." Molecular and Cellular Probes. 1998. 12, 301-308

[7] Vojdani, A., et al. "Detection of Mycoplasma Genus and Mycoplasma Fermentans by PCR in Patients with Chronic Fatigue Syndrome." Immunology and Medical Microbiology, 1998

[8] Nicolson, Garth L., et al. "Mycoplasmal Infections in Chronic Illnesses: Fibromyalgia and Chronic Fatigue Syndromes, Gulf War Illness, HIV-Aids and Rheumatoid Arthritis." Medical Sentinel. Volume 4, Number 5. September/October, 1999

[9] Nicolson, Garth, et al. IBID

[10] Cox, IM, et al. "Red Blood Cell Magnesium and Chronic Fatigue Syndrome." Lancet. 1991;337:757

[11] Romano, TJ, et al. "Magnesium Deficiency in Fibromyalgia Syndrome." J. Nutr Med. 1994;4:165

[12] Evengard, B et al. "Cerebral Spinal Fluid Vitamin B12 Deficiency in Chronic Fatigue Syndrome." Proceedings of the American Association for Chronic Fatigue Syndrome Research Conference; 1996

[13] Regland, B et al. "Increased Concentrations of Homocysteine in the Cerebrospinal Fluid in Patients with Fibromyalgia and chronic Fatigue Syndrome." Scandinavian Journal of Rheumatology 1997, 26: 301

Chapter 4

Natural Hormones
Part I

Natural Hormones Part I

It is nearly impossible to treat chronic illness or achieve optimum health without first ensuring that the hormonal system is properly functioning. The hormonal system in many of my patients who suffer with chronic disorders such as arthritis is often in disarray.

Hormones are chemical substances, produced from glands in the body, which have a specific regulatory effect on the activity of the body. Hormones control all of the physiological reactions in the body. Life itself is not possible without hormones.

Hormones have anti-aging effects and healing properties in the body. In those who suffer from a chronic illness such as arthritis, it is difficult for the body to properly heal injured tissues without an adequately functioning hormonal system.

My experience has shown that those with a chronic illness will have very low hormone levels. These depressed hormone levels inhibit the body's natural production of chemicals necessary for healing. In addition, these low levels of hormones prevent the immune system from optimally functioning. The use of synthetic hormones (e.g., Provera and others) can further exacerbate the situation.

Hormones work in the body in a lock-and-key fashion. After the hormone is released from the gland, it travels through the blood stream and binds to a receptor in a cell of the body. The hormone would be analogous to the key and the receptor would be similar to the lock. After the hormone (i.e., the key) binds to its receptor (i.e., the lock), a chemical reaction occurs in the body.

Synthetic Hormones Versus Natural Hormones

There are two categories of hormones that can be used to treat a hormonal imbalance: natural hormones (e.g., natural progesterone) and synthetic hormones (e.g., Provera).

A natural hormone is a substance generally made from a plant product, which has the same chemical structure as the body's own hormone. In other words, the body cannot distinguish the shape of its own hormone from the natural plant-derived version. Examples of natural hormones include natural progesterone, natural estrogens, DHEA, natural testosterone, natural hydrocortisone and human growth hormone. More information on natural hormones can be found in my book, The Miracle of Natural Hormones, 2nd Edition.

Figure 1: A Comparison of a Natural Hormone (Natural Progesterone) and a Synthetic Hormone (Provera)

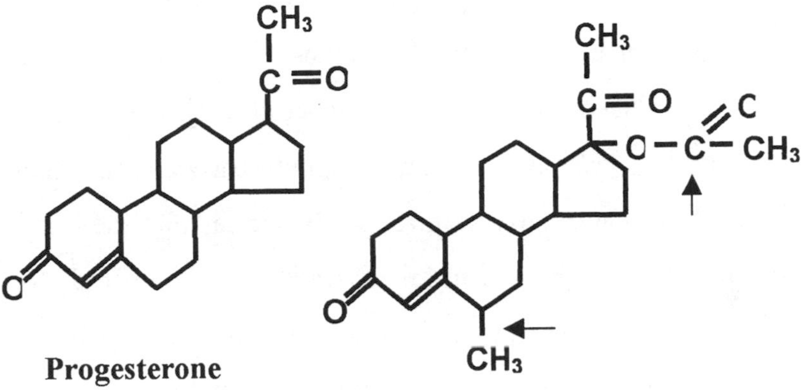

Progesterone

Provera

The difference between the natural hormone, progesterone, and the synthetic version, Provera, is illustrated in this diagram. The arrows in the Provera illustration point out the additional side chains added to progesterone. These added chains make Provera a foreign substance in the body, leading to an increased risk of adverse effects.

Synthetic hormones are man-made products that have been chemically altered. Examples of synthetic hormones include Synthroid, Levothroid, Provera and Prednisone. A synthetic hormone does not have the same structure as the hormone produced in the body. (See Figure 1 for a comparison of a synthetic hormone, (Provera), and a natural hormone, (natural progesterone.) Because synthetic hormones have an altered shape, they will not bind to the body's receptors in exactly the same way that a natural version of the hormone will. This altered binding of a synthetic hormone makes it a foreign substance to the body and will result in an increased risk of adverse effects and decreased efficacy as compared to natural hormones.

It has been my clinical experience that synthetic hormones do not work as well as their natural counterparts and that they are more likely to cause adverse effects. It is clear that the body will more readily accept a natural hormone as compared to the synthetic version. Therefore, I recommend that natural hormones should be used in all cases that require hormonal therapy. Natural hormones are safer and work better than their synthetic counterparts every time.

Thyroid

This chapter will review the importance of ensuring an optimally functioning thyroid gland. Chapter 5 will discuss DHEA, natural testosterone, natural hydrocortisone, natural progesterone and human growth hormone.

The thyroid gland is a butterfly-shaped gland located in the lower part of the neck. Though it weighs less than an ounce, the thyroid gland is responsible for many critical functions in the body.

Every single muscle, organ and cell in the body depends on adequate thyroid hormone levels for optimal functioning. I have found that even a slight deficiency of thyroid hormone, a condition known as hypothyroidism, can tremendously impact one's health. It has been my experience that those who have a chronic illness, such as arthritis, will often have a hypothyroid condition. In fact, I have found it nearly impossible for these individuals to overcome their illness without also addressing a hypothyroid condition. (See Table 3, page 72 for more information on the signs of hypothyroidism.)

Natural thyroid hormone, known as Armour Thyroid is much more effective in treating hypothyroidism than are synthetic versions such as Synthroid and Levothroid. Although Armour Thyroid does not exactly mimic the human body's production of thyroid hormone, it is the closest derivative of human thyroid hormone currently available.

The symptoms of hypothyroidism are listed in Table 3. A diagnosis of hypothyroidism should not be made solely on blood tests, as is primarily done in conventional medicine. An accurate diagnosis should encompass correlating the blood tests along with basal temperatures (Table 4, page 79) and with physical exam signs and symptoms. This is a truly a holistic way to diagnose a thyroid problem. My experience has shown that relying solely on blood tests to make the diagnosis of hypothyroidism will miss approximately 30-40% of the cases. All of the patients mentioned in the case studies below had thyroid blood tests performed before treatment. Occasionally, thyroid blood tests do not correlate with other signs of hypothyroidism. This will be more fully discussed in the Discussion section.

Table 3: Symptoms of Hypothyroidism

The symptoms of hypothyroidism include the following: fatigue, difficulty getting up in the morning, cold extremities and intolerance to cold, dry skin, psoriasis, eczema, acne, arthritis, recurrent infections, constipation, menstrual disorders, premenstrual syndrome (PMS), infertility, hypercholesterol, arteriosclerosis (i.e., heart disease), obesity and difficulty losing weight, hypoglycemia, diminished sweating, brittle nails, poor memory, depression, headaches and migraine headaches, fibrocystic breast disease, ovarian cysts, and weakness.

Case Studies

Roberta, 45 years old, had been diagnosed with Lupus at age 34. "I was devastated at the diagnosis. I had been feeling very fatigued for years before my doctor was able to make a diagnosis. When I look back on it, I am sure the fatigue was related to the Lupus," she stated. Roberta started developing arthritic pain shortly before her diagnosis was made. "I felt like an old lady. I would wake up stiff as a board, and I could barely move my hands." She was initially treated with steroids that provided relief from the pain, but she could not tolerate the side effects. "The treatment was worse than the illness," she claimed. Roberta's pain was somewhat controlled with nonsteroidal anti-inflammatory drugs (e.g., Motrin), but she could not overcome the fatigue. Roberta's condition left her unable to hold a job, and she had difficulty doing her daily activities. When I first met Roberta, she had many signs of hypothyroidism. She had a puffy face, poor eyebrow growth, dry skin, a thickened tongue and cold extremities. I diagnosed Roberta with hypothyroidism and started her on Armour Thyroid hormone (a natural thyroid preparation explained in the Discussion section). Roberta immediately felt more energetic. "I felt as if a cloud had been lifted off me. My brain started working again, and my energy started to return." Now, two years after beginning treatment for hypothyroidism, Roberta is able to work part-time. Her fatigue is completely gone, and she feels like a new person.

Fatigue is often the first symptom one will exhibit before a diagnosis of a chronic illness, such as Lupus, is made. Fatigue is also a cardinal sign of hypothyroidism. It has been my observation that a large percentage of those with chronic illnesses (e.g., Lupus, arthritis, fibromyalgia) have a poorly functioning thyroid gland, and they often exhibit significant improvement in their condition when treated for hypothyroidism.

Sam, age 61, was suffering from a severe case of rheumatoid arthritis (RA). His hands were swollen and painful to touch. "You know Doc, my brain feels young; but my body feels old," he said. Sam had been diagnosed with RA five years before. He had been treated with Placquenil (a disease-modifying anti-rheumatic drug or DMARD) and Methotrexate. Sam did feel some improvement from the medications, but the arthritis continued to progress. He complained of always feeling cold and especially of having cold hands and feet. "My hands turn blue when I go outside in the cold," Sam claimed. He was also very constipated and had a very high cholesterol level. He lamented, "I eat great and I can't get that cholesterol level down." Sam had a very low basal body temperature, and thyroid tests indicated a hypothyroid condition. Upon taking Armour Thyroid and the antibiotic Minocin (see Chapter 2), the swelling in his fingers immediately went down. Furthermore, Sam's constipation was resolved and his cholesterol fell dramatically, without any further changes in his diet. "I can't believe how much better my arthritis is. I was able to cut my medications (Placquenil and Methotrexate) in half," Sam commented.

Constipation, high cholesterol levels and cold extremities are common signs of a hypothyroid condition. I have found that combining thyroid treatment with other treatments, in this case with the antibiotic Minocin, provides a better response than does using the treatments individually. All of the treatments covered in this book are synergistic with one another. In treating chronic illness, the best results are often achieved by combining therapies. In Sam's case, the combination of Armour Thyroid with Minocin proved extremely beneficial.

Discussion

The thyroid gland produces approximately one teaspoon of thyroid hormone per year. Even a small variation in the production of thyroid hormone will have a tremendous impact on the body. When the thyroid gland does not produce enough thyroid hormone, signs of hypothyroidism will be present. (See Table 3 for many of the signs of hypothyroidism.)

The thyroid gland produces a hormone, Thyroxine, commonly known as T4. T4 is an inactive form of thyroid hormone in the body. In order for T4 to be activated in the body, it is converted to a more active hormone, Triiodothyronine, known as T3. T3 is the "activated" form of thyroid hormone that exerts its influence on all the cells in the body. (See Figure 2, below.)

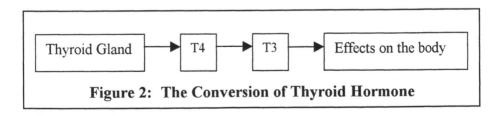

Figure 2: The Conversion of Thyroid Hormone

My experience has shown that those with a chronic disorder will not effectively convert T4 to T3, consequently exhibiting many of the signs and symptoms of hypothyroidism. There are many reasons why the body cannot effectively convert thyroid hormone to its more active form:

1. Deficiencies of trace elements such as selenium, iodine, iron and zinc
2. Medications such as beta-blockers, Dilantin, theophylline and chemotherapeutic agents
3. Low-protein and low-fat diets
4. Toxins such as mercury, pesticides and alcohol
5. Hormonal imbalances in the body (e.g., adrenal imbalances)

The TSH Test

Presently, the most common blood test used by doctors to diagnose a thyroid disorder is the TSH (thyroid stimulating hormone) test. The TSH test primarily reflects circulating T4 levels in the body. Since T3 is the more active thyroid hormone affecting the body (i.e., increasing metabolism, producing heat, etc), solely relying on the TSH test to diagnose a hypothyroid condition will result in missing many of those who have hypothyroidism.

David Derry, M.D., Ph.D., a thyroid expert and researcher from British Columbia asks, "Why are we following a test (i.e., the TSH test) which has no correlation with clinical presentation?" He feels that relying solely on the TSH test to make the diagnosis of hypothyroidism will miss many individuals suffering from the consequences of hypothyroidism. "The TSH test needs to be scrapped and medical students taught again how to clinically recognize low thyroid conditions," claims Dr. Derry.[1] Dr. Derry feels chronic fatigue syndrome and fibromyalgia are both conditions which result from untreated hypothyroidism. He points out that shortly after the medical community began using the TSH test to diagnose hypothyroidism, the signs and symptoms of chronic fatigue and fibromyalgia began to be described in the medical literature. Dr. Derry feels the signs and symptoms of chronic fatigue and fibromyalgia are one way a low thyroid condition can be expressed.

Many conditions, such as nutrient deficiencies, are thought to block the thyroid hormone at the cellular level, thus producing a clinically low thyroid state with normal blood indices. All too often physicians rely solely on laboratory work to make the diagnosis, often ignoring the patients' clinical condition, (being fatigued, being cold, etc). A wise physician in medical school once told me, "The patients will always tell you their diagnosis, if you'll listen to them. You should never rely solely on the lab to make the diagnosis." I believe there would be a lot less untreated hypothyroidism if physicians heeded this advice today. Dr. Gerald Levy, an endocrinologist and chief of medicine at the University of Pittsburgh School of Medicine, feels that there are many unknown factors which affect conventional testing, including drugs and disease states. His opinion is that hypothyroidism is a subtle disease and that it can be easily missed by conventional testing.[2]

A recent article in the British Medical Journal called into question the idea of relying solely on blood tests to confirm a diagnosis of hypothyroidism. The author of the study claims, "Experience has shown that thyroid function tests, like all the signs and symptoms associated with hypothyroidism and hyperthyroidism, are not totally reliable. The fact that the clinical aspects of assessing thyroid dysfunction are being sidelined is a cause for concern. Doing more tests will lead to further confusion."[3]

It has been my experience that many of my patients will have normal blood tests for thyroid function; yet they exhibit many of the signs and symptoms of hypothyroidism. This is particularly true in those who suffer from a chronic illness (such as arthritis, fibromyalgia or chronic fatigue). In fact, it is well known that thyroid function tests are often inaccurate during a systemic illness.

How To Diagnose Hypothyroidism

One measure of how the thyroid is functioning is through monitoring the basal body temperatures. A basal body temperature is the temperature taken first thing in the morning while lying in bed. Table 4 shows how to check your basal body temperature.

The thyroid is responsible for the body's metabolism and the production of heat. Hypothyroid individuals will often report being cold or having cold hands and feet. By checking the basal temperature, one can gather information on how the thyroid is performing. Generally, a low basal temperature (<97.8 degrees Fahrenheit) may indicate a hypothyroid state.

Table 4: How To Check Your Basal Body Temperature

1. Shake down a basal thermometer the night before and place it at your bedside.

2. Upon awakening, place the thermometer snugly in your armpit for a period of ten minutes and record your temperature for five days in a row. You must not get out of bed before checking your temperature, or you will have an altered temperature.

3. For women who are menstruating, the temperature should be taken on the second day of menstruation. This is the best time in a woman's menstrual cycle to get an accurate basal temperature. For men and postmenopausal women, it makes no difference when the temperatures are taken.

Dr. Broda O. Barnes, a pioneer in the diagnosis and treatment of hypothyroidism, found that the basal body temperature was one indicator of thyroid function. The basal body temperature is one measure of the metabolic state of the body. In a low metabolic state, which is often seen in hypothyroidism, the body's temperature will often be low. A low basal body temperature (<97.8 degrees Fahrenheit) may reflect a hypothyroid state. I have found that following basal body temperatures is a very helpful test for diagnosing and treating hypothyroidism.

As part of a complete examination, thyroid blood tests should be measured. These include the following:

1. TSH
2. T4 Total
3. T3 Total

Thyroid function is best determined by correlating one's health history, clinical examination, conventional blood testing and serial monitoring of basal temperatures. This is truly a holistic and complete way to diagnose a thyroid disorder. As previously mentioned, I believe that relying solely on blood testing may miss up to 40% of those with thyroid problems. Conventional physicians often ignore the complaints of a patient if the blood tests for thyroid function indicate normal values. I have evaluated and treated many patients for hypothyroidism who have normal blood test results. Many times these patients had every clinical sign present to make a diagnosis of hypothyroidism (cold hands and feet, fatigue, headaches, high cholesterol levels and others). These clinical signs were correlated with low basal body temperatures, which in hypothyroid individuals will typically run below 97.4 degrees Fahrenheit. Most of these patients will improve almost immediately on small amounts of Armour thyroid hormone. In addition, their basal temperature will increase into the normal range of 97.8-98.2 degrees Fahrenheit.

A recent study showed that simply checking the TSH levels revealed that thirteen million Americans might have an undiagnosed thyroid problem.[4] I believe this number would be significantly higher if the researchers had taken into account the history, physical exam signs and the basal temperatures.

I have found that those with a chronic disorder, such as arthritis, will often have a hypothyroid condition. Furthermore, as previously stated, I have found it nearly impossible for these individuals to overcome their chronic condition unless the thyroid condition is appropriately diagnosed and treated.

Treatment

For treatment of hypothyroidism, I recommend using natural thyroid hormone, most commonly known as Armour Thyroid, instead of synthetic thyroid preparations such as Synthroid and L-Thyroxine. Armour Thyroid is a porcine thyroid preparation, containing both T4 and T3 in proportions very close to the natural human thyroid output. It also has other factors that allow the conversion of T4 to the active form T3 to occur more readily. Synthetic thyroid preparations, such as Synthroid or L-Thyroxine, contain only T4 thyroid hormone, which must be converted to T3 in order to be effective. Many individuals, especially those with a chronic illness, will be unable to fully convert T4 to T3. Therefore, they will respond much better to a natural preparation such as Armour Thyroid, rather than synthetic versions such as Synthroid, since Armour Thyroid converts more readily to the active thyroid hormone T-3.

Final Thoughts

A complete discussion on hypothyroidism is beyond the scope of this book. There are also many environmental (e.g., toxins) and nutritional factors that may impact the thyroid gland. For more detailed information I refer the reader to my book, The Miracle of Natural Hormones 2nd Edition.

It is imperative to insure a properly functioning thyroid gland in order to overcome illness and achieve optimum health. I recommend that you work with a health care provider who is knowledgeable about the items I have outlined in this chapter in order to get an accurate diagnosis of hypothyroidism and to begin the proper treatment of hypothyroidism. The Barnes Foundation is an organization that was created to carry on the work of Dr. Broda O. Barnes. The Barnes Foundation can recommend a physician who can work with you. The Foundation can be reached at the following address:

Broda O. Barnes, M.D. Research Foundation
P.O. Box 98
Trumball, CT 06611
(203) 261-2101
www.brodabarnes.org

[1] Derry, David. Letter to British Medical Journal, 10/17/99

[2]"Hypothyroidism: a treacherous masquerader." Acute Care Medicine, May,

1984

[3] O'Reilly, Denis. "Thyroid Function Tests- Time for a Reassessment." British
Medical Journal, 5/13/2000; 320:1332-1334

[4] Canaris, Gay, et al. "The Colorado Thyroid Disease Prevalence Study." Arch.
Intern. Med. Vol. 160, 2/28/2000.

Chapter 5

Natural Hormones
Part II

Natural Hormones Part II

This chapter will further add to the discussion in Chapter 4 about the clinical effectiveness of using natural hormones to promote health and treat disease. Chapter 4 reviewed the benefits of natural thyroid hormone. This chapter will focus on the benefits of using other natural hormones; DHEA, natural testosterone, natural hydrocortisone, natural progesterone and human growth hormone.

As previously mentioned, natural hormones are substances derived from natural sources, which have the same chemical structure as the body's own hormones. Natural hormones can be used to effectively treat chronic conditions such as arthritis, fibromyalgia and others.

It is well known that hormone levels decline as we age. An example is shown in the graph of aging and declining DHEA levels on page 89. Does aging cause the hormone levels to fall or are the falling hormone levels responsible for the signs and diseases associated with aging? I do not have the answer, but I have found that using small amounts of natural hormones is effective for slowing down many of the signs of aging, including muscle loss, weakness, mental decline, wrinkling and others.

I have also observed that those with a chronic disease will often have lower levels of hormones than will healthy individuals of the same age. For example, nearly all of my patients with rheumatoid arthritis have significantly depressed hormone levels, particularly DHEA and testosterone levels. In fact, most of the people suffering from any chronic disorder will have suppressed hormone levels. Furthermore, the more ill one is, the further depressed the levels.

Again a question can be asked: Are the suppressed hormone levels responsible for the illness or does the illness result in suppressed hormone levels? I do not have a definitive answer to this question either, but my experience has shown that the proper use of natural hormones in conjunction with diet and nutritional support (Diet -- Chapter 6 and Nutritional Support -- Chapter 9) can result in a patient overcoming chronic conditions such as arthritis, fibromyalgia, chronic fatigue syndrome and other autoimmune disorders.

I believe that a well functioning hormonal system is necessary to promote health and to promote healing reactions in the body. This can be accomplished only with the use of natural hormones. Synthetic hormones do not work as well, nor do they promote true healing reactions in the body. For more information on the clinical use of natural hormones, I refer the reader to my book, The Miracle of Natural Hormones, 2nd Edition.

DHEA

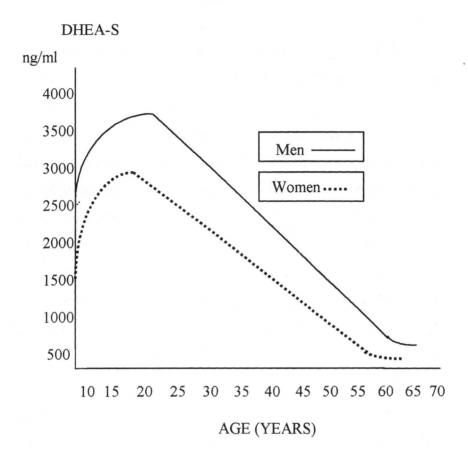

FIGURE 3: DHEA levels and the age-related decline. [1]

DHEA is an adrenal hormone. The adrenal glands are located at the upper pole of the kidneys. DHEA is an acronym for Dehydroepiandrosterone. DHEA levels, like the other hormone levels in the body, peak at a young age and fade throughout life. (See Figure 3.) Furthermore, I have observed consistently low DHEA levels in elderly patients as well as most individuals suffering from a chronic disease such as Lupus, Crohn's, ulcerative colitis, fibromyalgia, chronic fatigue syndrome, rheumatoid arthritis or multiple sclerosis.

In prolonged stressful states, the adrenal glands may under-function and produce sub-optimal levels of their hormones, including DHEA and other adrenal hormones. The adrenal hormones DHEA and testosterone are known as anabolic (i.e., tissue building) hormones. When the body has been injured, adequate amounts of the anabolic hormones are necessary for the tissue to heal. William Jeffries, a professor of endocrinology at Case Western Reserve University, has published numerous articles and books describing how the body will have a difficult time healing when the levels of the adrenal hormones are inadequate. He recommends using small amounts of the adrenal hormones to aid the body in healing.[2] My clinical experience validates Dr. Jeffries' findings.

In my practice, I have found that close to 100% of patients with autoimmune disorders (such as Crohn's, ulcerative colitis, Lupus, multiple sclerosis, rheumatoid arthritis, fibromyalgia and others) have significantly depressed DHEA levels. In addition, most of these patients show clinical improvement in their condition upon using physiologic (i.e., small) replacement doses of DHEA. Others have reported similar positive results with using DHEA to treat chronic conditions.[3]

There have been several studies that show that DHEA levels are depressed in patients with autoimmune diseases. One study on patients suffering from severe Lupus was conducted at Stanford University and showed that DHEA supplementation improved the patients' disease state as well as reduced their need for high dose steroids.[4]

Case Study: DHEA

Patricia, at age 48, had been suffering from rheumatoid arthritis for ten years. "It has taken over my life. My hands are swollen and ache every morning, and some mornings I have difficulty getting out of bed," she lamented. Patricia had to take a non-steroidal anti-inflammatory drug on a daily basis to help relieve the pain. "The medicine rips up my stomach, but I have to take it or I am in constant pain. I feel as if I am an old lady already. I have no energy to do anything," said Patricia. When I examined Patricia, I noticed she had very poor muscle tone. Upon checking her serum hormone levels, I found that her DHEA-S level was very suppressed (360ng/dl). Upon taking 5mg of DHEA per day (in conjunction with some dietary changes: a gluten-free diet and supplement therapies), Patricia made a remarkable recovery; and her DHEA-S level improved to a healthy 1750ng/dl. "Within two weeks of beginning the DHEA, I noticed an immediate improvement. The swelling began to go down, and my energy began to increase. I started to feel like my old self again," she reported. Patricia has been on DHEA for over two years, and she is now able to exercise (yoga) and do volunteer work. Patricia was also treated with other natural hormones, including natural thyroid hormone and natural testosterone. She has regained all of the energy she felt was missing, and her arthritic pain has subsided. "I get aches and pains now like anyone else; however, the joint pains I used to have are gone. I am just thrilled," she said.

As previously mentioned, I find most of my patients who have an autoimmune disorder will have low DHEA levels. In most cases (as in Patricia's case), significant improvement will be noted when DHEA is taken as part of a holistic program of dietary changes and nutritional supplementation.

DHEA Dosage and Recommendations

DHEA levels should be investigated in all people who have a chronic illness. However, the reader should be aware of differences in the reported normal ranges of different laboratories. I have found that adequate levels of DHEA necessary to overcome illness for men range from 2,000-3,000ng/dl and for women, from 1,500-2,500ng/dl. All levels in this book are measured as the sulfate form of DHEA, DHEA-S. These levels closely approximate the peak levels of DHEA seen in Figure 3. In treating chronic illness, I have often found it necessary to raise DHEA levels to approximate the peak levels mentioned above.

DHEA levels should be measured before supplementation with DHEA and should be checked at routine intervals in order to optimize the dose. I recommend pharmaceutical grade DHEA made by a compounding pharmacist. I have often found that DHEA sold over-the-counter at health food stores is not reliable. DHEA should be taken on an empty stomach for better absorption. DHEA works best in small amounts (men: 5-10mg/day and women: 2-8mg/day) and has synergistic effects with the other natural hormones covered in this book. Because of the synergistic effect of taking DHEA with the other natural hormones, I rarely use DHEA as the sole hormone to treat illness or to promote the health of the individual.

Side Effects: DHEA

Side effects from using physiologic doses of DHEA are rare. The side effects I have witnessed have been acne and moodiness, occurring in approximately 5% of my patients, usually young females. I have also noticed very mild hair growth occurring in

1% of my patients, a problem that is easily managed with reducing the dose.

Natural Testosterone

Natural testosterone, when used prudently, is a very important part of hormone balancing in both men and women. Testosterone is one of the major regulators of sugar, fat and protein metabolism in the body. Testosterone is the main hormone produced by the testicles in men, with smaller amounts produced by the adrenal glands. In women, testosterone is produced in the ovaries and the adrenal glands. Women produce testosterone in much smaller amounts than men.

There are two forms of testosterone supplementation currently available: natural testosterone and synthetic testosterone. Natural testosterone is made from plant products and has the same chemical structure as testosterone that is produced in the human body. I have found natural testosterone to be very safe and effective in treating many different conditions, including autoimmune disorders. I believe natural testosterone, rather than a synthetic version, should be used in all cases of testosterone therapy.

Case Studies: Natural Testosterone

Jackie, age 47, had been diagnosed with Lupus at the age of 35. She reported symptoms of joint and muscle pain, muscle wasting, difficulty concentrating and always feeling an overwhelming fatigue. "I just feel like I am slowly wasting away," she claimed. Her physician was treating her with Prednisone, a synthetic steroid hormone. Her testosterone level was so low it was not even measurable in my lab. Upon taking 5mg of natural testosterone, she noticed an improvement in all of the above symptoms. "I feel so much better. I definitely have a higher energy level and I even look younger," she claimed. Her testosterone level improved to a healthy .7 ng/ml, with normal levels for women ranging from .3-.8ng/ml. Jackie was also found to be hypothyroid and to have low levels of progesterone and DHEA. She noted improvement when treated with each of these natural hormones. In addition, I treated her with nutritional supplements. One and one-half years later, she feels her disease has stopped progressing and may actually be reversing itself. Furthermore, she has been able to stay off all high dose steroid treatments, thus avoiding the negative side effects associated with steroids (osteoporosis, weight gain, etc).

I have yet to see a patient ill from Lupus or another autoimmune disease that does not have significantly depressed testosterone and DHEA levels. Furthermore, these patients often have lowered thyroid and ovarian function. Most people suffering from autoimmune disorders will respond favorably to physiologic replacement of natural hormones.

Patricia, recalled from the DHEA case study on Page 91, was initially treated with DHEA. This treatment resulted in a *marked improvement in her rheumatoid arthritic condition. Patricia was also found to have a severely low testosterone level. It was so low that it was reported by the laboratory as < .2ng/ml (i.e., not measurable). Patricia had many of the signs of a low testosterone level, including a very poor libido. "My husband is incredibly frustrated with me. I have absolutely no interest in having intercourse. It used to be such an important part of my life and now it is the farthest thing from my mind," she said. In addition, Patricia had many of the signs of muscle loss on the initial physical exam. Upon taking a small amount of natural testosterone (3mg/day), Patricia noticed an improvement in her libido. After one month of taking natural testosterone, she claimed, "My husband wants to thank you. I feel alive again, almost youthful. Our sex life is beginning to get back to normal. My husband now wants to come in and see you and have his levels checked." Furthermore, the declining muscle mass that Patricia was experiencing reversed itself within three months.*

There is no question that natural testosterone can improve a declining libido in men and women. I have found sub-optimal testosterone levels in my patients who suffer from chronic disorders such as arthritis. Testosterone, like DHEA, is an anabolic (i.e., muscle building) hormone that aids the body in repairing injured tissues in many chronic disorders such as arthritis.

Discussion: Natural Testosterone

As illustrated in Patricia's and Jackie's cases, it has been my experience that most people with immune system disorders (i.e., autoimmune disorders) have severely depleted testosterone levels. One study found that the use of testosterone significantly improved the symptoms in patients with Lupus. The authors of this study concluded that low levels of androgens, which include testosterone and DHEA were thought to play a role in the development of autoimmune disease.[5]

My experience has shown that most patients who are ill from an autoimmune disease, such as rheumatoid arthritis or Lupus, have depressed levels of testosterone. These patients generally respond favorably to small amounts of natural hormones, including natural testosterone.

The discussion of testosterone brings thoughts of huge body builders artificially taking anabolic (i.e., muscle and tissue building) steroids in order to bulk up. When taken in extremely large doses, testosterone does promote the growth of huge muscles and can even result in aggressive and violent behavior. In addition, large doses of testosterone can lead to the development of hypertension, baldness, acne and other deleterious side effects.

However, with physiologic replacement doses--small doses that will not shut off the body's own production of the hormone--these negative side effects will not occur. In fact, I have found testosterone supplementation to be one of the most beneficial hormone replacement treatments for men and for women.

As with the other hormones mentioned in this book, I recommend using the natural form of the hormone: in this case, natural testosterone. My reasoning is the same as previously presented. In order to get the maximum benefit from hormonal replacement therapy, it is important to try and mimic the body's own production of its hormones. When used appropriately, I have found natural testosterone to be extremely safe and effective, without any appreciable adverse effects. This safety record is contrasted with the use of the synthetic form of testosterone (methyl testosterone or testosterone enanthinate), which is primarily used in the United States. Methyl testosterone (a synthetic version of testosterone) has been found to be carcinogenic.[6]

Natural testosterone is also effective for treating a wide range of disorders, as shown in Table 5. Dr. Jonathan Wright, one of the pioneers of using natural hormones to promote optimum health, describes in his book, Maximize Your Vitality and Potency for Men Over 40 (Smart Publications) the positive results he has encountered with the use of natural testosterone.

Natural Testosterone Dosages and Recommendations

When supplementing with testosterone, I recommend only natural testosterone (not the synthetic derivatives of testosterone) because it more closely mimics the body's own production of testosterone. Doses for women usually average 2-10mg/day. For men, doses usually range from 40-120mg/day. I prefer to use testosterone in cream form, as it is well absorbed through the skin. I recommend USP grade, micronized natural testosterone, which can easily be made by a compounding pharmacist. For more information on finding a compounding pharmacist, please see Appendix B.

Table 5: Benefits of Natural Testosterone

The benefits of replacement doses of testosterone are truly amazing. These include improving osteoporosis, improving the symptoms of diabetes, increasing a general sense of well being and improving libido and sexual functioning. In addition, testosterone can decrease negative mood parameters including those of anger, irritability, nervousness, and tiredness.[7] Testosterone has been shown to prevent and treat coronary artery disease and to improve and treat autoimmune disorders such as Lupus and rheumatoid arthritis. It has also been shown to be able to rejuvenate muscle mass.

Side Effects: Natural Testosterone

Doses of testosterone that are too high can lead to the development of hypertension, acne, hair loss, anger, and mood swings. I have not observed any major negative effects in the use of physiologic replacement doses of natural testosterone. There is some concern that testosterone could adversely affect prostate cancer. Consequently, I do not recommend testosterone therapy for a patient who has had a diagnosis of prostate cancer. Taking an herb, saw palmetto (300mg twice per day), may block any possible negative effect of testosterone on the prostate by stopping the conversion of testosterone to dihydrotestosterone. Dihydrotestosterone is thought to cause the excess growth of the prostate gland.

Natural Progesterone

Progesterone is one of two major hormones produced by the ovaries in females. (The other is estrogen.) Progesterone is primarily produced in the second half of the woman's menstrual cycle and is the hormone necessary for the survival of the fetus.

Men produce very tiny amounts of progesterone in the adrenal glands and the testicular glands. In men and women, a small amount of progesterone is produced in the adrenal glands, where it acts as a precursor for the adrenal estrogens, testosterone, and cortical steroids (cortisol). There are two types of progesterone currently available: natural progesterone and synthetic progesterone (e.g., Provera). Natural progesterone is made from plant products and has the same chemical structure as the progesterone produced in the human body. For a comparison of the difference in the chemical structure of natural progesterone and Provera, see Figure 1, page 69. I have found natural progesterone to be much more effective and safer for treating illness and promoting health than synthetic forms of progesterone, such as Provera.

Case Studies and Discussion

At the age of 45, Roberta (recalled from Chapter 4) was suffering from Lupus. I treated her initially with natural thyroid hormone, and she noticed a significant improvement in her condition. When I added natural progesterone to her regimen, she continued to improve. "I used to have PMS and heavy bleeding with my periods. Since starting the natural progesterone, all of my PMS symptoms are gone and I now have normal periods with a manageable amount of bleeding. Taking natural progesterone has significantly improved my life," she happily reported to me.

I have treated hundreds of women who suffer from PMS with natural progesterone. I believe PMS is a cardinal sign of a progesterone deficiency. Roberta's progesterone level was checked on the twentieth day of her cycle; it was extremely low at 9ng/ml. (Normal levels should be 20-30ng/ml.) It is rare to find a woman suffering from PMS who does not have an extremely low progesterone level. As in Roberta's case, heavy menstrual bleeding is another sign of a progesterone imbalance that can often be reversed by using a small amount of natural progesterone.

Natural Progesterone Doses and Recommendations

Natural progesterone is available in a cream form, which is absorbed through the skin, and in a pill form. I usually recommend using the cream because its absorption appears to be better than that of the pill. There are several natural progesterone creams available in health food stores. My research has shown, however, that many over-the-counter brands of natural progesterone are not consistent: the strengths can vary from jar to jar. I have found better results with U.S.P. grade micronized progesterone, typically derived from soybeans and formulated by a compounding pharmacist. I use strengths from 2-10%, applied directly to the skin. Progesterone levels improve with this method; and, most importantly, symptoms improve. I recommend using natural progesterone the last two weeks of a menstrual cycle and for three weeks of the month in a postmenopausal woman.

Side Effects: Progesterone

The side effects for natural progesterone that I have observed include breast tenderness, moodiness and weight gain. These side effects are very rare and are usually dose related. These are contrasted with the adverse effects from the synthetic version of progesterone (Provera). The side effects from Provera include breast cancer, blood clots, fluid retention, breast tenderness, nausea, insomnia, depression and others. I have yet to observe a serious side effect with the use of natural progesterone. In discussions with colleagues who also use natural progesterone, they also report very few adverse effects.

Final Thoughts: Natural Progesterone

I believe Provera is a very toxic drug. A recent study in the <u>Journal of the American Medical Association</u> showed that the use of synthetic progesterone (Provera, Depo-Provera and others) increased the risk of breast cancer by 800% as compared to the use of estrogen alone.[8] Synthetic progesterone drugs should not be used for any condition. Natural progesterone should be used for all cases of progesterone therapy.

Natural Hydrocortisone

Hydrocortisone is a hormone produced in the adrenal glands--the same glands that produce DHEA. Adequate production of hydrocortisone is the body's major line of defense against stressful situations, including infections and injuries. In a stressful situation, one of the body's primary responses is an increase in the output of hydrocortisone. Without this increased production of hydrocortisone, the body is unable to adapt to the stressful situation.

When there is not an adequate production of hydrocortisone, there is an increased susceptibility to illness (such as the common cold and other infectious processes) as well as longer recovery times and more severe infections from illness. In fact, adequate levels of hydrocortisone are necessary for the immune system to function properly and for the body to heal itself from illness or infection.

For people who have deficient hydrocortisone production, physiologic replacement doses (i.e., small doses) can improve the immune system as well as reverse many chronic conditions without any serious side effects. These positive effects cannot be achieved with the high doses (i.e., pharmacologic doses) commonly employed in conventional medicine.

In individuals who suffer from chronic illness, I have found it absolutely necessary to properly evaluate the adrenal glands by measuring their output of hydrocortisone. It is impossible to effectively treat many arthritic disorders (rheumatoid arthritis, scleroderma, Lupus and others) without ensuring adequate functioning of the adrenal glands. Measuring hydrocortisone levels can determine whether the adrenal glands are functioning properly. Treatment with small doses of natural hydrocortisone (Cortef), when indicated, has proven to be invaluable in helping these patients overcome their illness. Other disorders that can be treated with physiologic (i.e., small) doses of hydrocortisone, when indicated, include chronic fatigue syndrome and fibromyalgia.

Case Studies: Hydrocortisone

Julie, age 44, had been diagnosed with scleroderma two years previously. Scleroderma is classified as an autoimmune disorder in which the connective tissue (including the skin, heart, lungs and other organs) becomes hard and rigid. Arthritic symptoms often develop with this disorder. "I first noticed pain in my hips and my knees. The pain would move all around my body. At first, the Motrin prescribed by my doctor gave me some relief, but after a while it stopped working," she claimed. Julie had to quit working as a schoolteacher because she did not have enough energy to get through the day. "My symptoms continued to worsen," she said. "I became so tired I could not read a book. I had to take a nap during the day because I was so tired. The pain in my joints kept getting worse, and I began to gain weight even though I was not eating any differently." When Julie developed esophagitis (an inflammation of the esophagus), she was diagnosed with scleroderma. "I was devastated. My doctor could not tell me why I was sick, and he could not offer me an effective treatment. I thought I was going to die," she lamented. I found Julie to have a hypoadrenal condition (i.e., a low output of the adrenal gland hormones). Julie was appropriately placed on a small amount of natural hydrocortisone (Cortef: 5mg, three times per day). "It was amazing. Taking this small amount of a medication provided me with a lot of relief. My joints did not hurt as much, and I began to get my energy back," she happily stated. In addition, Julie was treated with DHEA and natural progesterone (both are adrenal hormones) and natural thyroid hormone. I prescribed a daily regimen of supplements (vitamins B-12, B-6, and E as well as selenium and flax seed oil). Finally, Julie was found to have a mycoplasma infection (see Chapter 2), and the antibiotic Minocin was added to her treatment program. "It has now been two years since I started this treatment program. I feel 95% better. What little pain I now have usually goes away with an aspirin. My energy and my weight are also back to normal. My rheumatologist tells me there is no cure for scleroderma. He is wrong. I feel I have cured this illness," she said.

I have found that scleroderma and the various other autoimmune disorders have many common factors. Most of these conditions place a terrible strain on the hormonal glands of the body, particularly the adrenal glands. Small (i.e., physiologic) doses of the adrenal hormones are necessary for the body to overcome these illnesses as well as to promote healing. In addition, these hormones work best when combined with other hormones, such as thyroid hormone, when indicated. This is a holistic way to approach these complicated and serious illnesses.

I have also found that many of those suffering from autoimmune disorders have an underlying bacterial infection, such as mycoplasma. These patients will not fully improve until this condition is appropriately diagnosed and treated. (For more information on the infectious nature of these and other illnesses, see Chapter 2.)

Natural Hydrocortisone Dosages and Recommendations

The possible side effects associated with hydrocortisone and other steroids include the promotion of weight gain, osteoporosis, arteriosclerosis and blood sugar abnormalities. However, I have observed no major side effects with the use of hydrocortisone in physiologic replacement doses--doses less than 40mg per day. The main side effect I have observed with taking a physiologic dose is a small weight gain, usually less than five pounds. Usually this weight gain will subside after one or two months of taking hydrocortisone.

Human Growth Hormone

Human growth hormone is secreted by the pituitary gland, which is located in the center of the brain. It is named human growth hormone because its production peaks during the intense growth spurt of adolescence. Children lacking the proper production of human growth hormone will have an extremely short stature. Adults lacking human growth hormone have many signs of accelerated aging (increased skin wrinkling, decreased energy levels, poor sexual function, increased body fat and signs of osteoporosis). Furthermore, accelerated cardiovascular diseases are common in adults with human growth hormone insufficiency. I have found that people who suffer from arthritis and other chronic disorders often have severely depressed levels of growth hormone.

After the pituitary secretes human growth hormone, it causes the liver to secrete another hormone called insulin-like growth factor 1 or IGF-1 as illustrated in Figure 4. It is IGF-1 that

Pituitary Gland $\longrightarrow$ Growth Hormone $\longrightarrow$ Liver $\longrightarrow$ IGF-1

Figure 4: The release of human growth hormone from the pituitary, which leads to the release of IGF-1 from the liver.

is responsible for the effects of human growth hormone on the body. IGF-1 is easily measured in the blood and is the most common measurement used to assess growth hormone status. All levels of growth hormone mentioned in this book are measured as IGF-1 levels.

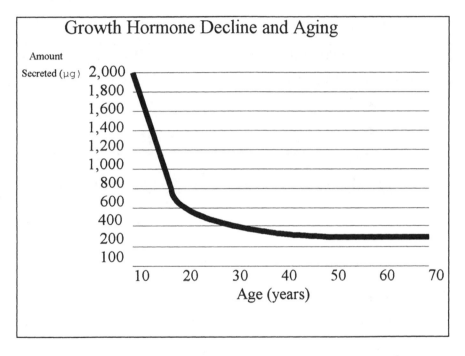

Figure 5: Human growth hormone decline as related to aging[9]

In adults, human growth hormone production gradually declines as one ages, as is illustrated in Figure 5. This gradual decline parallels the age-related decline of DHEA and testosterone. After the age of twenty, human growth hormone levels fall by 50% approximately every seven years. It is clear that those who suffer from a chronic illness will have suppressed levels of growth

109

hormone (and often all of the hormones produced in the body). Perhaps by raising levels of human growth hormone (as well as DHEA, testosterone and the other hormones) to levels present at younger years, we can slow down or even reverse many of the signs and symptoms of aging and lesson the symptoms of such chronic diseases such as arthritis, chronic fatigue syndrome, fibromyalgia and many others. Supplementation of human growth hormone does appear to clinically reverse many of the signs of aging in most people who take it.

Diagnosing a Deficiency of Human Growth Hormone

Human growth hormone levels can be adequately tested in the blood. I utilize IGF-1 as a good measure of growth hormone levels. I have found that effective serum levels for IGF-1 range from 200 to 300ng/ml in men and women.

Case Study: Growth Hormone

At the age of 57, Rene (recalled from Chapter 2) had experienced significant improvement in the symptoms of Vasculitis with the use of antibiotic therapy. Though Rene felt much better, there was still room for improvement. Upon checking a growth hormone level (i.e., IGF-1), I found her level was low at 90ng/ml. (Normal level is 200-300ng/ml.) Rene was also experiencing many of the signs of advanced aging. "I feel like I have aged tremendously since I became ill. Though I feel better, my muscles are very weak and I have a very difficult time maintaining muscle tone," she said. After taking a small amount of growth hormone (0.05U/day), Rene noticed an immediate improvement. "My strength began to return almost immediately. I couldn't believe the difference growth hormone made. I was able to exercise longer, and my mind felt sharper," she claimed. Rene's growth hormone level increased to 209ng/ml. Rene continues to use growth hormone today, and she still shows signs of improvement in her condition.

I have found physiologic doses of human growth hormone to be safe and effective in promoting health, reversing the signs of aging and helping patients overcome illness.

The downside of the use of growth hormone is the expense: it can cost over $2,000 per year. How do you raise growth hormone levels without using growth hormone? Exercise has been shown in numerous studies to enhance the body's natural release of human growth hormone. I have also found that the use of physiologic doses of other natural hormones (natural thyroid hormone, natural testosterone, DHEA, melatonin and others) can increase growth hormone levels. Nutritional supplementation with amino acids has also been shown to raise growth hormone levels.

In a study (to be published) that I conducted, an interesting nutritional product, Gammanol Forte (manufactured by Biotics Research: 1-800-437-1298), was shown to raise growth hormone levels by over 45% in women.

Growth Hormone Dosages and Recommendations

Human growth hormone is given in injectable form. It is given in doses of 0.05-1.5 I.U. per day in a subcutaneous injection, which is similar to an insulin injection. It is best given in two divided shots per day, usually in the morning and at bedtime; this mimics the body's own rhythm of secreting growth hormone. Growth hormone, like all the other hormones mentioned in this book, should be used in physiologic (i.e. small) doses only. It can be measured in the blood as an IGF-1 test. I have found effective serum levels for IGF-1 range from 200-300ng/ml.

Side Effects: Growth Hormone

One side effect of using human growth hormone is increasing the risk of acromegaly. Acromegaly is a condition where huge amounts of human growth hormone are secreted in the body resulting in a higher incidence of cardiac problems and premature death. Acromegaly is seen in athletes who take massive doses of human growth hormone and in other people who are born with a pituitary gland that erroneously secretes excess amounts of human growth hormone. I have not experienced any signs of acromegaly with the use of physiologic doses of human growth hormone.

Other adverse effects of human growth hormone include carpal tunnel syndrome, achiness in the joints and muscles, and edema. These side effects have been reported with high doses of human growth hormone and are almost nonexistent when using lower doses. Most of these side effects are easily reversible by lowering the dose. I have observed few adverse effects with the use of physiologic doses of human growth hormone.

Final Thoughts

Natural hormones are very effective and safe when used appropriately. A proper hormonal evaluation should be undertaken for everyone who suffers from a chronic illness. Physiologic (small) doses of natural hormones should be employed to treat deficiencies. There is little reason to use synthetic versions of hormones when there are natural versions available. A natural product will work better in the body and have fewer adverse effects than a synthetic product every time. However, natural hormones should not be used without close monitoring by a qualified health care practitioner skilled in their use. "The concept of replacing hormones with identical hormones in the correct proportions at the correct time makes obvious sense," writes Dr. Jonathan Wright in his book, <u>Natural Hormone Replacement For Women Over 45</u> (Smart Publications). I recommend Dr. Wright's book for further information on natural hormones.

Furthermore, I believe in using natural hormones prepared by a compounding pharmacist rather than over-the-counter products because the compounded preparations are of a superior quality and contain consistent doses. To find a compounding pharmacist in your area contact the International Academy of Compounding Pharmacists at:

IACP
P.O. Box 1365
Sugar Land, Texas 77847
(800) 9227-4227
www.compassnet.com/iacp

[1] Whitaker, Julian. Dr. Whitaker's Guide to Natural Hormone Replacement. Phillips Publishing, Inc., Potomac, Md, 1996. Reprinted with permission. Readers may call 1-800-539-8219 for more information or to subscribe to Dr. Whitaker's newsletter, Health and Healing.

[2] Jeffries, William. Safe Uses of Cortisol. Thomas. 1996.

[3] Claebrese Vp et al. "DHEA in multiple sclerosis: positive effects on the fatigue syndrome in a non-randomized study." In Kalimi M. Regelson W. The Biological Role of Dehydroepiandrosterone. De Gruyter. New York. 1990. p. 95-100

[4] Van Vollenhovenm, Ronald. Arthritis and Rheumatism. September, 1994; 37(9); 1305-10

[5] Lahita, RG. "Increased oxidation of testosterone in systemic Lupus erythemaosis." Arhtritis Rheum. 1983;26:1517-1521

[6] Nutrition and Healing Newsletter, Vol. II No. 12, 1995

[7] Wang, C, et al. "Testosterone replacement therapy improves mood in hypogonadal men- a clinical research center study." Journal of Clinical Endocrinologic Metabolism. 1996;81:3578-83

[8] Journal of the American Medical Association. January 26, 2000; 283:485-491

[9] Journal of NIH Research, Adapted from, April, 1995

Chapter 6

Diet

Diet

This section of the book was written to assist the reader in using proper dietary techniques that will allow the body to overcome illness and will provide the body with the proper nutrient levels for achieving optimum health.

A balanced diet is essential in order to achieve optimum health and to overcome a chronic illness such as arthritis. Sadly, most Americans eat a poor diet. An improper diet will not only result in a poorly functioning immune system, it will also inhibit the natural healing mechanisms of the body, promote obesity and accelerate the aging process.

Food consists of three major macronutrients: carbohydrates, protein and fat. Carbohydrates are found in plant products and include starches and sugars. They are found in fruits, vegetables, grains, pasta, bread, cookies, alcohol, etc. Proteins are the building blocks of the body and they form the muscles and organs of the body. An adequate intake of protein is also necessary to produce hormones. Sources of protein include animal products (the most complete form of protein), vegetables such as beans and legumes, and seeds and nuts. Fat contains more energy than either protein or carbohydrates, and it is essential for forming cell membranes and for hormone production. In addition, fat acts as a carrier for fat-soluble vitamins, including Vitamins A, D, E and K. Fat is found in animal and vegetable products. Vegetable fats are found in oils such as olive oil, flaxseed oil, corn oil, etc.

The American public has been told by organizations such as The American Medical Association, The American Cancer Society, dieticians, their own physicians and the government that we must eat low fat, high carbohydrate foods in order to be healthy. This is expressed in the food pyramid that is so well known. I refer to this diet as the "Standard American Diet" or the SAD diet (because it leads to poor health and SADness).

In the last twenty years fat consumption has decreased by 11% in this country. What has been the result of twenty years of following a diet low in fat and high in carbohydrates? It has made Americans the most obese people on this planet. In fact, during the last twenty years while fat intake has decreased, obesity has increased by 32%.[1] In addition, the incidence of chronic illness has accelerated during this same time frame.

The Standard American Diet is a major cause of the tremendous growth of degenerative disorders seen in this country. These disorders include arthritis, autoimmune disorders, cancer, coronary artery disease and many others. Also, this diet promotes an imbalanced hormonal system. In order to promote health, we must understand the important role of food in providing fuel and nutrients for our bodies. We can now also understand how to use food to provide our bodies with essential nutrients to promote true healing.

One of the first steps in promoting health and healing is looking at food as a drug. Dr. Barry Sears, author of the bestseller Enter the Zone, claims, "Food is the most powerful drug we will encounter."[2] Proper choices of food will provide the body with the raw materials necessary to promote health, along with supporting a healthy immune system. Sadly, a healthy immune system is nearly impossible to maintain while eating the typical American diet. In fact, the people I see in my practice that eat a low fat, low protein, high carbohydrate diet often have the most severe illnesses and have a difficult time achieving optimum health. Often, those suffering with a chronic illness such as arthritis are following the wrong dietary plan, one that is increasing the severity of their condition.

In order to allow the body to overcome a chronic illness such as arthritis, one needs to eat a balanced diet by combining the proper amounts of protein, fats and carbohydrates. A balanced diet can provide the body with the proper nutrients necessary to have a healthy immune system, which in turn, promotes healing in the body. The proper nutrients come from all food sources—proteins, fats and carbohydrates.

Protein

Protein is the second most common substance in our bodies (second only to water). Adequate protein intake is necessary to promote general health and a balanced hormonal system. Proteins are the building blocks for all of the structural tissue of our bodies and are required to form the muscles, bones, nerves, arteries, veins and skin.

Hormones are synthesized from protein. Enzymes, the catalysts for physiological reactions, are also made from protein. Enzymes are found in raw food products such as fruits, vegetables and animal products and are deactivated at temperatures above 118 degrees Fahrenheit. Enzymes in food aid our body's digestive processes. Therefore, it is important to eat adequate amounts of raw food in order to achieve the benefits of natural enzymes.

Protein is found in animal products and in vegetables. Free-range eggs (eggs from un-caged chickens that are not fed any hormones or antibiotics) are a wonderful source of protein and should be eaten on a daily basis. Animal protein is the only source of complete protein available (i.e. containing all of the essential and non-essential amino acids). Vegetable protein, found in seeds, nuts, legumes and cereals, does not contain all of the essential amino acids.

The typical American diet recommends limiting animal products (consequently limiting protein) and increasing the consumption of grains and vegetables. Protein deficient individuals cannot satisfy the body's daily needs for maintaining structure and repairing injuries. Therefore, protein deficient individuals have an increased chance for developing a degenerative disease such as arthritis. These individuals may also have hormonal deficiencies (with the thyroid being the most affected gland). Protein deficiency can also promote vitamin and mineral deficiencies (in particular, Vitamin B-12 deficiency).

Vegetarians must take special care to be certain that their diet is appropriately balanced with all of the essential and non-essential amino acids. Historically, humans have eaten animal products, augmented with vegetables, fruits and nuts. It is my belief that eating organic animal products (those that are free of antibiotics and hormones) is a safe and healthy way to provide the body with the necessary elements (protein and fat) to promote health and to have a properly functioning immune and hormonal system. My experience has shown that those who limit protein intake are more likely to develop degenerative disorders.

Fat

Fat is the most maligned macronutrient. Sally Fallon, author of Nourishing Traditions writes, "Protein cannot be adequately utilized without dietary fats. That is why protein and fats occur together in eggs, milk, fish and meats."[3] We have been brainwashed by the dieticians and the diet industry into believing that eating fat is bad for our health and that dietary fat is responsible for obesity. However, many studies indicate that low-fat diets do not improve health or curb obesity.

In the United States, from 1910 to 1970, saturated animal

fat consumption decreased from 83% to 62% of the American diet. During this same time, heart disease (as well as degenerative diseases such as cancer, autoimmune disorders and arthritis) increased over 1000% in Americans.[4] Low-fat diets not only contribute to poor health; they also guarantee a poorly functioning hormonal system and a weakened immune system.

Not all fats are created equal. Many physicians and dieticians consider all fats to be a problem. However, eating the right kind of fat (one which is rich in nutrients) is essential to having a healthy immune system and is necessary for the body to overcome illness.

Fats are found in most natural foods. Fat is an essential nutrient for our body and is necessary for the following functions:

1. Energy production
2. Forming the skin and coverings of the major organs of the body
3. Maintaining cell integrity in every cell in the body

Fats can be classified as organic substances that are insoluble in water. All fats can be classified according to their chemical structure. The following are the most common fats in our diets:

1. Monounsaturated fats (e.g., olive oil)
2. Saturated fats (e.g., animal fats, butter, coconut oil)

3. Polyunsaturated fats (e.g., flaxseed oil, fish oils, most vegetable oils)

Fats, like all substances, can have good and bad properties. "Good" fats provide the body with healing nutrients and help the cells of the body maintain their integrity. They are found in whole foods and are necessary for healing and the promotion of optimal health. "Bad" fats poison the cells of the body and cause nutrient deficiencies, particularly deficiencies of the fat-soluble vitamins A, D, E and K. "Bad" fats are found in hydrogenated oils and trans fatty acids.

Fat is found in both animal and vegetables sources. Fat has a higher energy content than either proteins or carbohydrates. Every cell membrane in the body contains fat, and all steroidal hormones are produced from the fat-like substance cholesterol. Fat is necessary for the absorption of fat-soluble vitamins, including Vitamins A, D, E and K. Protein cannot be adequately utilized without proper amounts of fat in the diet.

Since fat is so important to our over-all health, it is crucial that we obtain a sufficient amount of the proper types of fat. Ingesting the wrong types of fat will increase the chance of developing a degenerative condition such as arthritis. A very low-fat diet or a diet high in the wrong types of fat will promote a poor immune system, a poor healing capacity and a malfunctioning hormonal system.

Essential Fatty Acids

Fats can be further classified into essential fatty acids and non-essential fatty acids. Unsaturated fatty acids are termed essential fatty acids because our bodies cannot manufacture them; therefore, they must be taken in from the diet. Essential fatty acids consist of omega-3 fatty acids (derived from linolenic acid) and omega-6 fatty acids (derived from linoleic acid). Essential fatty acids are necessary for a wide range of functions in the body, including hormone production and immune system functioning. A deficiency of essential fatty acids has disastrous consequences on the functioning of the immune system. The immune system cells are dependant on receiving adequate amounts of essential fatty acids from the diet.

Deficiencies in essential fatty acids have been linked to many chronic, degenerative disorders, including coronary artery disease, hypertension, hormone abnormalities, autoimmune disorders, strokes and cancer. Unfortunately, the Standard American Diet is deficient in omega-3 fatty acids. Adequate amounts of omega-3 fatty acids are found in free-range eggs, cold-water fish (non-farm raised), some vegetable oils (flaxseed oil is one of the best sources) and some nuts and seeds. For most people, it is important to increase the amounts of omega-3 fatty acids in the diet.

Another concern with essential fatty acids is the disproportionately large amount of omega-6 fatty acids relative to omega-3 fatty acids found in the typical American diet, which can lead to obesity and an increase in inflammatory diseases. Omega-6 fatty acids are found in most vegetable oils (e.g., sunflower, safflower, corn, primrose, borage and black currant oil) and many nuts and seeds.

Cooking oils are a major source of fat in our diet. Using the wrong type of cooking oil can have a disastrous effect on our health. The cooking oil used by the majority of Americans not only contains the wrong kind of fatty acid but also is devoid of almost all nutrients. The vegetable oils commonly found in grocery stores have been processed into partially hydrogenated vegetable oils, which results in the removal of almost all of the nutrients from the oil. Also, these processed oils may contain the heavy metal nickel, which is used in the hydrogenation process.

The hydrogenation process of oils also causes the oil to contain large amounts of trans fatty acids, which are known toxins to the body. These oils are damaging to the body's DNA and are associated with many degenerative diseases including cancer, arthritis, heart disease, diabetes, obesity, immune system disorders and others.

Partially hydrogenated vegetable oils are found in margarine and in many other oils such as corn oil, canola oil, and cottonseed oil. Margarine should be avoided at all costs; butter should be the spread of choice.

Every cell membrane in our body contains a mixture of unsaturated and saturated fatty acids. These fatty acids give the cell membrane its fluidity and flexibility. The cell membrane is the point where nutrients are absorbed into the cell. Ingesting the wrong types of fatty acids forces the body to accumulate the wrong types of fatty acids into each of the cells of the body. When we eat hydrogenated fats containing trans fatty acids, these toxic substances are actually incorporated into our cell membranes. The cells can no longer absorb nutrients and perform the critical functions necessary to promote health.

Dr. Walter Willet, chairman of the nutrition department at the Harvard School of Public Health, claims, "Introducing trans fatty acids into the American diet is the single most harmful thing the food industry has done in the last 100 years."[5] In addition, Dr. Willet estimates that consumption of trans fatty acids in the United States accounts for thirty thousand premature deaths per year.[6]

Partially hydrogenated oils are toxic to the body and should not be used under any circumstances. Furthermore, those with a chronic illness must make a special effort to eliminate these toxic substances from the body. Many products are made with partially hydrogenated oils; these include crackers, cookies, cakes, pasta, and bread. Whenever you see that partially hydrogenated oils have been used in a product, avoid it. It is impossible for the body to overcome a chronic illness when ingesting the wrong types of fat.

On the contrary, using the right cooking oil can have significant health benefits. Good oils are generally found in darkened containers because light is damaging to healthy oils. They should have an expiration date, as contrasted with hydrogenated oils that are devoid of all living matter and can sit on the shelf forever. Healthy cooking oils include extra virgin olive oil and coconut oil.

Despite the fact that the nutrition experts consider coconut oil atherogenic (i.e., promoting coronary artery disease), it is a good source of saturated fatty acids, especially for vegetarians who eat little saturated fat. Saturated fats are necessary for the proper utilization of essential fatty acids. Coconut oil is commonly used by populations in the tropics where there is little heart disease. Choosing the right oil can have a major impact on the immune system, hormonal system and over-all health.

In addition to healthy oils, organic nuts and seeds are healthful sources of fats. Also, good sources of fat are organic animal products, including eggs, meat and chicken. Organic animal products have a much more favorable fatty acid composition than do the products of conventionally raised animals.

Carbohydrates

Carbohydrates are produced in all green plants in the form of starches and sugars. Glucose and fructose are examples of sugars. Starches are sugar molecules bound together. Carbohydrates are necessary for the body to transform fat into energy. However, the body has mechanisms to convert excess carbohydrates into fat. Sadly, the Standard American Diet contains too many carbohydrates and has made Americans the most obese people on the planet.

There are two categories of carbohydrates: refined and unrefined. Refined carbohydrates are formed from the processing of foods, a process which strips food of many of its vitamin and mineral components. The following are examples of ingredients and foods that contain refined carbohydrates:

1. White sugar and white flour
2. Pasta
3. Corn starch
4. Breakfast cereals
5. Cookies, cakes, bagels, doughnuts and other baked goods

Eating these "refined" foods is very damaging to the body. Since these foods lack vitamins, minerals and enzymes, which are necessary for proper digestion, the body must use its own source of vitamins, minerals and enzymes. Overuse of refined carbohydrates can lead to a multitude of health problems, including obesity and nutritional deficiencies. In addition, the increase in the use of refined carbohydrates has been directly associated with the rise in degenerative disorders (arthritis, diabetes, cancer, autoimmune disorders, fibromyalgia, chronic fatigue and others) in the industrialized world over the last fifty years.

Refined carbohydrates also interfere with normal blood sugar regulation in the body. Refined carbohydrates are absorbed in the body very quickly and will result in a rapid rise in blood sugar levels. The pancreas will respond to this rise in blood sugar levels by raising insulin levels. Excess insulin levels are an oxidant stress on the body and will accelerate any chronic disease process. Elevated insulin levels also deplete the body of a chemical called Cyclic AMP. Hormone synthesis in the body depends on adequate Cyclic AMP levels. The rapid rise in blood sugar levels coupled with a rapid rise in insulin levels will result in insulin insensitivity and, ultimately, diabetes. Also, this rapid rise in blood sugar levels will lead to poorly functioning immune and hormonal systems.

Unrefined carbohydrates are found in whole foods, such as fruits, vegetables and whole grains. These whole foods contain vitamins, minerals, enzymes and fiber that aid the body in their digestion. Therefore, the body does not become depleted from the ingestion of unrefined carbohydrates (in contrast to the ingestion of refined carbohydrates).

One must choose carbohydrates that do not excessively raise blood sugar levels. Dr. Barry Sears, the author of The Zone books states, "All carbohydrates are not created equal."[7] Carbohydrates can be rated on a "glycemic index" scale. Good carbohydrates will have a low glycemic index rating: they do not excessively raise blood sugar levels. "Bad" carbohydrates will have a high glycemic index rating: they will cause blood sugar to elevate quickly, resulting in an exaggerated insulin response. (A table listing the glycemic index of various carbohydrates is found in Appendix A.) There is no question that eating foods with a low glycemic index is more beneficial than eating foods with a high glycemic index.

Putting It All Together

So what do you do to give your body the best chance to heal itself and to achieve optimum health? I have found that a balanced diet containing adequate amounts of good sources of each of the macronutrients (i.e., proteins, fats and carbohydrates) will provide the body with the essential elements it needs to repair injured tissue, maintain a properly functioning hormonal system and promote a healthy immune system.

It is absolutely necessary to eliminate the excess use of refined carbohydrates (refined sugar and refined flour) in the diet. These substances deplete the body of its own source of vitamins and minerals, resulting in hormonal imbalances and causing a large oxidant stress on the body. I have found that limiting carbohydrates to no more than 40% of the caloric intake is paramount to this balancing regimen. In addition, adequate amounts of the right kinds of fat and protein (approximately 30% each of the total caloric intake) will allow the body to maintain good health. This combination parallels Dr. Sears' Zone diet. Although I do not agree with Dr. Sears on all points, I believe his books will provide readers with a good starting point for balancing their dietary regimen. For more detailed discussion of this topic, I refer the reader to two sources: Dr. Barry Sears' Enter The Zone and Sally Fallon's Nourishing Traditions.

Finally, I encourage the readers to think about the foods they are eating. We all need to take responsibility for the foods that we eat. If we eat foods that are devoid of nutrients (e.g., refined sugar), our health will suffer. Making simple dietary adjustments, including eliminating refined sugar and trans fatty acids and eating low glycemic carbohydrates, will result in an overall improvement in your health. If we eat whole foods that supply our bodies with good sources of nutrients, we will give our bodies the best chance to heal.

Case Study

Darlene, age 57, suffered with rheumatoid arthritis for fifteen years. "The pain in my joints only gets worse and worse. Every morning I wake up fatigued and stiff, and I can barely move my hands," she said. Darlene was being treated with Vioxx, an anti-inflammatory medication that gave her minimal relief. She had stopped eating red meat three years before, and she had adopted a very low protein diet. "Everything I read in the paper tells you that you should avoid red meat. I eat a lot of bread and pasta and very few animal products," she said. When I tested Darlene (with a serum blood analysis and a serum fatty acid analysis), I found her to be deficient in protein and fat. I told her to eliminate the trans fatty acids as well as all refined sugar from her diet, and to increase the good sources of protein and fat (whole foods, including nuts, seeds, legumes and organic animal products). When Darlene saw me for a recheck in six weeks, she could not believe the change in her condition. "Within a few days of changing my diet, my energy level began to rise," she claimed. "Here I was eating food that I thought was bad for me (organic eggs, red meat, nuts and seeds), and I immediately began to feel better. My joint pain and stiffness significantly improved. I no longer need to take the Vioxx every day. I can get by with using it a couple of days a week. I also couldn't believe the change in my weight -- I lost 5 pounds without even trying. That is the best part." Darlene was additionally treated with Minocin (see Chapter 2), natural thyroid hormone (see Chapter 4), DHEA (see Chapter 5) and vitamins and minerals. Today, Darlene feels that her condition is 90% improved. "My friends all ask me what I am doing since I look so much healthier," she said. "I tell them that I cleaned up my act and I am eating much healthier."

Final Thoughts

In my experience, the Standard American Diet, which consists of a low-fat, high-carbohydrate diet often leads to obesity and difficulty maintaining adequate hormone levels, as well as increasing the prevalence of chronic diseases. A recent study reported in <u>The Journal of the American Medical Association</u>

reported that although Americans have a relatively low consumption of animal fats and a low cholesterol concentration, the United States ranked second to last out of thirteen western countries studied for overall health.[8] This study is one more indication that the Standard American Diet is failing us and leading to increased disease.

The first step toward achieving and maintaining good health is to eat the right foods, including eating foods rich in the good sources of fat and protein. In addition, eating food in the proper amount and eliminating (or at least decreasing) trans fatty acids and refined sugar and flour from your diet is necessary to take the first steps toward finding your optimal health. A health care provider who is knowledgeable about proper nutrition can suggest a diet that is right for you. A good resource for finding a physician or nutritionist to guide you is the Price-Pottinger Nutritional Foundation (1-800-366-3748).

[1] Heini, Adriann, et al. " Divergent Trends in Obesity and Fat Intake Patterns: The American paradox." American Journal of Medicine. March, 1997. vol. 102:26.

[2] Sears, Barry. Enter the Zone. Harper Collins. 1995, p. 27.

[3] Fallon, Sally. Nourishing Traditions. Promotion Publishing, 1995.

[4] Fallon, Sally, IBID. p. 5.

[5] Consumer Reports, November 1998, p. 60

[6] Galland, Leo. Power Healing. Random House, 1997 p.156

[7] Sears, Barry. IBID. 1995, p. 71

[8] Starfield, Barbara. "Is U.S. Health Really the Best in the World?" JAMA, Vol. 284, No. 4. 7/26/00, p. 483

Chapter 7

Allergies

Allergies

This chapter was written to assist the reader in searching for safe and effective treatment strategies to aid the immune system. I have found that those who suffer with arthritis and related conditions such as fibromyalgia and chronic fatigue syndrome often have multiple allergies complicating their illness. It is unclear which comes first, the illness or the allergies. In either case, treating the allergies will often improve the functioning of the immune and hormonal systems and allow the body to begin to overcome disease.

An allergy can be defined as a "hypersensitive state acquired through exposure to a particular allergen, re-exposure bringing to light an altered capacity to react."[1] In simpler terms, an allergy is an inappropriate response of the immune system to a substance. These "allergic" substances can be anything: food, pollens, bee stings, dust, chemicals, perfumes, cigarette smoke, etc. Often a substance can be harmless to one person and cause a severe reaction in another. The Roman Philosopher Lucretius said, "What is food for some may be fierce poison for others."

The inappropriate response of the immune system can take many different forms: breathing difficulties (e.g., wheezing in asthmatics), runny nose and watery eyes, headaches, chest pain, arthritic pain, diarrhea, anxiety, fatigue and many others. Traditional allergists describe the immune system response as an IgE (Immunoglobulin E) related disorder. The theory is that the body produces antibodies to various substances that ultimately result in the release of chemical mediators, such as histamine, that cause the allergic symptoms (i.e., watery eyes, runny nose, wheezing, etc.)

Conventional approaches to allergy problems revolve around using drugs such as antihistamines and allergy shots. Antihistamines work by blocking the release of histamine from the cells of the body. Allergy shots work by blocking the body's inappropriate immune system response to the allergen. Allergy shots can be effective for some environmental allergies (trees, grass, weeds, dust, etc.), but they have not proven to be very effective for food allergies. My experience has shown that a large percentage of individuals who have a chronic illness also have food allergies.

Studies

The relation of food allergies to arthritis has been studied for over fifty years.[2] In one study, twenty-two patients with rheumatoid arthritis were given an allergy elimination diet (i.e., they were told to avoid many allergy-promoting foods). Ninety-one percent had improvement in their arthritic symptoms; and 86% found specific foods that worsened their condition, with grains and milk being the most common allergens.[3]

Other studies have also shown the relation of food allergies to arthritis.[4] [5] [6] [7] One study found that in seventy patients with rheumatoid arthritis who were treated with dietary modification, the following foods were found to cause arthritic symptoms:[8]

1. Corn: 56 %
2. Wheat: 54%
3. Pork: 39%
4. Oranges: 39%
5. Milk/Oats: 37%
6. Rye: 34%
7. Egg, Beef, Coffee: 32% (each)

When patients in the above study were given dietary modifications that included avoiding the offending foods, 19% did not require any medication after a follow-up period of one and one-half to five years.

It is imperative to evaluate any individual who is suffering from a chronic illness for food allergies. In my experience, the most common offending foods are grains and dairy products.

Often a trial of avoidance of these items (without any testing) is very effective at relieving many of the symptoms of arthritis.

Environmental allergies can also have an impact on one's health. An environmental allergy can be an allergy to almost anything: animals, pollens (trees, grass, weeds, etc.), chemicals, and others.

NAET

It is often necessary to do detective work to uncover the allergy or allergies that are impacting one's health. This may be accomplished by conventional allergy testing via skin tests. Also, there are blood tests that measure specific antibody levels in the blood. I have found an allergy elimination technique, NAET, to be very effective at diagnosing and treating food and environmental allergies.

NAET is named after its founder, Dr. Devi Nambudripod, and is an acronym for Nambudripod's Allergy Elimination Technique. This technique utilizes applied kinesiology and acupressure to diagnose and treat allergies. It is a safe, non-toxic, effective treatment program that I have used for over six years. A further discussion of NAET can be found later in this chapter.

Individuals with a chronic illness often have an allergic component to their condition. Many times their condition cannot be adequately treated until the allergies are properly diagnosed and treated. In the discussion section I will provide further information on how to diagnose and treat food allergies.

Case Studies

Hetty, age 59, suffered a downward spiral in her health over a ten-year period. "I was diagnosed with fibromyalgia ten years ago. I was working in a dental office, and I became very ill from exposure to the chemicals being used. At first, my brain became foggy; then my immune system went crazy. All the muscles of my body began to hurt, and I lost all of my energy. I had to stop working a short time after I became ill, and I basically became an invalid," she said. Hetty had a difficult time coming to see me. She missed her first three visits because she mixed up the days of the appointments. When she finally came for the office visit, Hetty told me that she felt like she was dying. She had become increasingly allergic to many foods, and she had a difficult time taking any vitamins. She stated, "Every time I try to take vitamins and minerals, my body aches and I can't think. I don't even know what to eat anymore. How am I supposed to get better if I can't eat good foods and if most vitamins and minerals make me sick?" When I first saw Hetty, she looked very tired. She was unable to work because of her condition. Using NAET, I diagnosed Hetty with allergies to many common foods, including milk, wheat, eggs and sugar. When the allergies were treated with NAET, Hetty felt an immediate improvement. "I couldn't believe the change. It was as if I started waking up again. I could start eating different foods again, and I began to regain my strength," she said. However, Hetty had the greatest improvement in her health condition when she was treated for an allergy to chemicals commonly found in a dental office: Nitrous Oxide and Fluoroethane. Immediately after the treatments for these items, Hetty's health took a dramatic turn. She regained her energy level, and most of the fibromyalgia pain disappeared. "NAET saved my life. I could not function before my allergies were diagnosed and treated. I feel like I have been given my life back," she claimed. Hetty was so thrilled with the improvement in her health that she became trained as a NAET practitioner. Presently, Hetty works in my office doing NAET treatments. She also takes a small amount of natural thyroid hormone (for hypothyroidism) and a small amount of DHEA.

As mentioned before, in patients suffering from a chronic illness and allergies, often it is difficult to distinguish whether the allergy or the illness comes first. In either case, significant improvement in health can be seen when allergy treatments are used concurrently with other modalities. In Hetty's case, I used NAET to treat her allergies while simultaneously treating her hypothyroidism with natural thyroid hormone. As previously mentioned, I have found that combining holistic treatments is much more effective than using the treatments individually.

George, age 48, had suffered with rheumatoid arthritis for five years. "One day I woke up and my joints started hurting. Since that day, I have never felt good. My hands always ache, and my fingers will swell for no reason," he said. I treated George with the antibiotic Minocin (see Chapter 2), and he began improving. He said, "When I started the antibiotic, I immediately got better. The swelling began to go down and the stiffness was much better." George found that his arthritis symptoms would worsen when he ate certain foods. "Every time I eat dairy products, I am swollen for a week. Even if a product has a little dairy in it, I will react to it," he claimed. Through NAET, I diagnosed George as having an allergy not only to dairy products but to calcium as well. "How can I be allergic to calcium? I thought my body needed calcium to help my bones," he said. I frequently find people with chronic disorders to be allergic (or sensitive) to various vitamins and minerals. Unless these allergies are fully cleared, the patients will often have a sub-optimal response to any therapy. George was cleared of an allergy to calcium and dairy products, and he immediately improved. "Within one day of the NAET treatment my energy level shot up, and my joint pain almost totally went away. Eating those foods containing calcium, as well as taking calcium pills, probably made my condition worse. All I know is that I feel tremendously better after going through NAET." George has continued receiving NAET treatments for various allergies and also continues to take Minocin, and his rheumatoid arthritis symptoms have completely resolved.

George's case again illustrates how the different treatment regimens can have synergistic effects. NAET was combined with the antibiotic therapy. Today, George remains symptom free, two years after starting treatment.

Grace, age 72, had found her chronic fatigue condition worsening over the past fifteen years. She said, "At first the fatigue was the only symptom I had. Then I started to become allergic to everything, including food. Now I can hardly eat anything. My diet is limited to brown rice and chicken." When I first met Grace, she looked pale and tired. A nutritional evaluation showed very low levels of vitamins and minerals in her body. She was deficient in many of the B vitamins as well as magnesium, calcium, zinc and other minerals. Grace was also anemic, with a low blood count and a low iron level. However, she was unable to take any supplements. "How can I take any supplements? They all make me sick. I get extremely tired and sick to my stomach when I take any vitamins or minerals," she said. Grace was also found to have a hypothyroid condition, but she could not tolerate taking any type of thyroid medication. After two months of NAET, her reactions to many foods began to subside. "It feels like a miracle," she claimed. "Foods that used to bother me, don't bother me at all. I am starting to feel so much stronger because I can eat again." In addition, Grace began to take her thyroid medication and noticed further improvement. "I feel like a new person. I can't remember when I had this much energy. My life has been given back to me. My husband is very thankful to have me back." Grace still receives periodic NAET treatments and continues to improve.

I have found NAET to be a wonderful tool for diagnosing and treating allergies, as is demonstrated by the case histories of

Hetty, George and Grace. NAET incorporates many different modalities: chiropractic, applied kinesiology, nutrition, and acupuncture. NAET is an effective, safe, natural way to help the body overcome illness.

How NAET Works

NAET works on the principal of energy flow. In acupuncture theory, health occurs when all of the energy circuits (i.e., meridians) of the body are open and functioning. In disease states, the energy centers are closed.

When the body comes in contact with anything (an odor, a food, a chemical, an article of clothing, etc), it must react to the substance. Our body reacts to these items in an energetic fashion. When the item is perceived as not harmful, the body's energy system will remain strong. If the item is perceived as harmful, there will be a drop in the body's energy system. Once the offending item is eliminated, the energy system will re-establish itself. Problems develop when the body is constantly exposed to offending items and cannot open up its energy centers, leading to serious health problems including immune system disorders.

NAET utilizes applied kinesiology to diagnose the problem and then uses acupressure to open up the body's energy system. It is an extremely simple yet effective technique for improving one's health. NAET, like acupuncture, facilitates the opening of blocked energy centers, which can then allow the body to maintain a healthy state. Though NAET is not helpful in all cases, it has been extremely successful in approximately 75% of my patients, helping them overcome many different allergies.

NAET should only be performed by those properly trained in the technique. To find a practitioner in your area you can call (714) 523-8900 or look on the NAET web site for practitioners at:

www.naet.com

Histamine-Allergy Connection

In an allergic state, the neurotransmitter histamine is frequently being released at high levels. There are only two natural substances that are known to lower histamine levels: water and salt. I find that many individuals who suffer from allergies are in a dehydrated condition and are deficient in salt. In most allergic conditions, symptoms can be improved by increasing water and salt intake. Salt and water can decrease the release of histamine from the mast cells of the body. In addition to treating those who suffer from allergies with NAET, I also recommend that each patient with allergies be evaluated (and if necessary treated) for a water and salt deficiency. Treatment with water and salt will be more fully explained in Chapter 8.

[1] Dorlands Illustrated Medical Dictionary. 26th Edition, 1981.

[2] Turnbull, JA. "Changes in sensitivity to allergenic foods in arthritis." Am. J. Dig. Dis. 1944; 11:182

[3] Hicklin, JA, et al. "The effect of diet in rheumatoid arthritis." Clin. Allergy. 1980;10:463

[4] Williams, R. "Rheumatoid arthritis and food: a case study." Br. Med. J. 1981;283:563

[5] Panush, RS, et al. "Food-induced arthritis. Inflammatory arthritis exacerbated by milk." Arthritis Rheum. 1986;29:220

[6] Zeller, M. "Rheumatoid arthritis: food allergy as a factor." Ann. Allergy 1949;7:200

[7] Mandell, M. et al. "The role of allergy in arthritis, rheumatism and associated polysymptomatic cerebro-viscero-somatic disorders: a double blind provocation test study." Ann Allergy 1980;44:51

[8] Darlington, L.G., "Dietary therapy for arthritis." Rheum. Dis. Clin. North. Am. 1991;17:273-285

Chapter 8

Water

Water

The human body is composed of 70-80% water, with the composition of the brain being closer to 85% water. Blood is 83% water, and muscles are 75% water. Because of this high concentration of water in the body, it is essential to have an adequate water intake to promote good health and optimal functioning of all of the cells. In fact, good health cannot be achieved without adequate water intake. In addition, proper amounts of salt need to be present along with the water in order for the body to be in a state of optimum health.

Dehydration acts as a tremendous stress on the body and is one of the major factors inhibiting the healing process. My experience has shown that almost all patients with a chronic disease will exhibit some signs of dehydration. In addition, all chronic diseases will be accelerated by inadequate water intake. For those who suffer with arthritis, it is impossible for the joints to heal without ensuring an adequate water and salt intake. In fact, one of the first signs of dehydration can be pain anywhere in the body, including the joint pain of arthritis.

F. Batmanghelidj, M.D. (a researcher and author on the benefits of water) states, "In a physically active part of the body that does not receive adequate water to wash away the toxic waste of metabolism, acidity will increase and at a certain point the nerve endings of the area will pass the information to the brain. The brain registers this chemical change as pain."[1]

Arthritic patients will frequently report pain in the joints of the body. Those with fibromyalgia report pain in the muscles of the body. Often, a common link between these two conditions is dehydration. In my experience, over 90% of patients who suffer from a chronic illness are dehydrated. Their condition will not improve until the dehydrated state is corrected, often with forced water intake. I recommend that dehydration be addressed before using vitamins, minerals, drugs, acupuncture or any other therapy.

Case Studies

At the age of 63, Carol had suffered with rheumatoid arthritis for over five years. She is a registered nurse who was thinking of retiring because of her illness. Carol was taking Motrin (a nonsteroidal anti-inflammatory drug) to help control the pain. She said, "Every morning I awaken tired, and it feels as if my joints are stuck in glue. It takes me over an hour just to get my hands to work. I can't stand the aching that goes along with the stiffness." When I first met Carol, she had many of the signs of dehydration. Her tongue was coated and appeared very dry. She had no skin elasticity. In addition, her nails had vertical ridges on them (one sign of a dehydrated state). After my examination of

Carol, I asked her to see me again in six weeks to review the tests that we had performed. The only suggestion that I gave her was to increase her daily intake of water. Carol was drinking only one glass of water per day, and she was drinking two to four cups of coffee and one soda per day. I asked her to increase her water intake to ten glasses of water, cut her coffee back to one cup and eliminate the soda. When Carol came back to see me in six weeks, she could not believe the results. She claimed, "Within ten days, I started to feel better. The first step was improvement in the joint stiffness. My mornings became so much easier. I did not have to fight with my body every morning just to get it to move. Also, my energy level began to pick up. I was definitely not as tired in the mornings." Carol reported her rheumatoid arthritis condition to be over 50% better just from drinking more water. "I was able to decrease by half the amount of Motrin I use. Some days, I wasn't using it at all. I could not believe that water could have that much of an impact on how I feel. I think I have been dehydrated my whole life," she said.

Joint stiffness (especially early morning stiffness) is one of the cardinal signs of dehydration. Water in the joints acts to flush out toxins and keep the joints lubricated. Inadequate amounts of water in the joints will produce stiffness and lead to arthritic changes over time.

Janice has been a nurse in my office for over ten years. When we began working together, I noticed Janice starting her day with a large mug of coffee. This mug would be refilled throughout

155

the day. In addition, at lunch, Janice would drink soda. Needless to say, this did not sit well with me. Janice developed back pain approximately three years ago. At first, it was just an annoyance; and then her symptoms worsened. "I started waking up every morning stiff as a board. I would have to stand in the shower for over ten minutes just to loosen up my back," she said. Janice would ask me to do manipulation to help her with her pain, but she would only get temporary relief from the manipulation. She said, "The adjustments would help for a day or two; then the stiffness and pain would come right back." During this time, I was encouraging Janice to drink more water. Her comment to me was, "I hate water. I feel sick when I drink water." One night, Janice had an acute spasm of her back and could not walk. She was taken to the emergency room where she had to be transported in a wheelchair. The doctor took x-rays of her back and told her she had arthritis and that she would need to take a month off of work and do physical therapy. In addition, he wanted to give her an IV of pain medication. Janice did not want any of these therapies. "I told the doctor that I would have to go home and start drinking water as my doctor (Dr. Brownstein) has been telling me. He looked at me like I was crazy when I told him I did not want the pain medication and to just get me some water. I started drinking water in the emergency room; after two glasses, the back pain started to ease a little bit. I continued to drink water the rest of that night, and the next day the back spasm and pain was 75% better. I could not believe it. I never went to physical therapy, and now I rarely experience any problems with my back." Janice also had other signs of dehydration, such as dry skin and eczema of her hands. "I thought my hands were dry because I wash them all the time at work. Now, my hands are smooth all of the time, even though I still wash my hands frequently throughout the day," she said. Janice has not had to have an adjustment of her spine since she increased her water intake two years ago.

Degenerative changes in the joints of the back (i.e., arthritis) will always be exaggerated by dehydration. The discs that support our back are made up of 75% water. Inadequate amounts of water will allow the discs to compress, causing pain and wearing of the joints and eventually leading to arthritic changes.

Back spasms and, in fact, muscle spasms anywhere in the body are almost always due (in part or in whole) to dehydration. My recommendations are to drink thirty-two ounces of water immediately after a spasm has started. It is rare that the spasm will not immediately improve when increasing the water intake, as was true in Janice's case.

Beverly, age 50, was diagnosed with fibromyalgia ten years before I saw her. She made a huge recovery from fibromyalgia when she began to exercise. "When I was diagnosed with fibromyalgia, I was miserable. I ached everywhere and I had difficulty sleeping. I vowed this was no way to live, so I decided to start exercising. I took up running and weight lifting. Not only did

I lose weight, but I began to feel better," she said. When I met Beverly, she had been exercising for six years. She felt that her fibromyalgia condition was 50% better. She was on Daypro, a prescription anti-inflammatory medication for pain, as well as the synthetic hormones Provera and Synthroid. Although Beverly was taking Synthroid, she had many of the symptoms of a hypothyroid condition, including very dry skin, thinning hair and constipation. I immediately changed Beverly to a natural thyroid hormone, Armour Thyroid (Chapter 4) and changed Provera to Natural Progesterone (Chapter 5). Through blood testing, I discovered that Beverly had high antibody levels of Mycoplasma bacterium. (See Chapter 2.) She was further treated with the antibiotic Minocin. I also found her to be dehydrated and recommended she increase her water intake. When Beverly implemented this program, she made an immediate improvement. Within two months of beginning this approach, most of her fibromyalgia problems went away. "It feels like a miracle," she said. "My head feels clearer, I hardly ache and I can exercise so much better. I feel like I have been reborn." Beverly recently went through a stressful period at home and stopped drinking water. She felt the difference in her health immediately. "When I wasn't drinking enough water, I couldn't exercise as well. My muscles felt like they were dead. My legs would hurt, and the body aches began to return. Also, I began to get headaches." When Beverly resumed drinking adequate amounts of water (for her, seventy ounces or more per day), all of these symptoms resolved.

I have found that fibromyalgia patients are almost always living in a chronically dehydrated state. Their condition generally improves when the dehydration is treated with water, as was demonstrated in Beverly's case.

Discussion

Water is an essential nutrient for everyone. Unfortunately, most people, especially those who suffer from a chronic illness, do not drink enough water; and this leads to more health problems. It is rare for me to see a patient with a chronic illness who does not have many of the signs of dehydration. The following are some of the signs of dehydration:

1. Fatigue
2. Dry tongue
3. Coated tongue
4. Vertical ridges on the nails
5. Dry skin
6. Poor skin elasticity

Many of the signs of aging, including the loss of elasticity of skin and muscles, are primarily due to the body's cells losing water. This water loss can be accelerated by many factors, including the following:

1. Inadequate water intake
2. Excess caffeine consumption
3. Excess soda consumption
4. Alcoholic beverages
5. Diuretic medication

The habitual over-consumption of sodas, coffee, tea and juice can lead to a chronic state of dehydration. Many people assume that by drinking beverages other than water, they are supplying the body with an adequate amount of water. This is not the case. These other liquids contain substances (e.g., caffeine, sugar and other solutes) that actually cause water loss in the body to accelerate. Caffeine is a potent diuretic. Chronic caffeine use can over-stimulate the adrenal glands and ultimately result in a depletion of the adrenal hormones. This can further exacerbate other hormonal irregularities and weaken the immune system. Another reason that dehydration is such a widespread problem in this country is the amount of soda consumed. A 1994 report of the beverage industry showed a per capita consumption of soda of 49.1 gallons per year!

Diuretic medications, often prescribed for hypertension, may also contribute to a dehydrated state. A study in Vienna that lasted over six years showed the potential danger of a dehydrated state. Men who drank five or more glasses of water per day had a 50% decreased risk of coronary artery disease as compared to men who drank less than two glasses of water per day. The men who drank the larger amount of water also had a 44% decrease in fatal strokes when compared to ones who drank little water.[2]

Since water is such a nourishing agent for the body, it is important to drink water in its purest form, without additives and chemicals. Bottled water contains chemicals leached from the plastic known as xenoestrogens. These chemicals can cause hormone irregularities. Tap water often contains chemicals (including fluoride and chlorine) harmful to the hormonal system and other substances that can contribute to health problems.

Fluoride is added to the water supply in many municipalities to help prevent cavities. However, fluoride is a known carcinogen, and the dose of fluoride necessary to prevent cavities has never been accurately determined. An article in Medical Hypothesis found the amount of fluoride commonly added to the water supply can damage immune system cells.[3] Dr. John Yiamouyiannis, one of the world's foremost authorities on the effects of fluoridation, states that fluoride, in the amount added to drinking water, "inhibits over 100 different enzymes in the cells of people living in fluoridated areas." His research (with the chief chemist at the National Cancer Institute) estimated that the fluoride added to the nation's water supply was responsible for 10,000 additional deaths from cancer per year.[4] A recent study in the journal Brain Research showed that low doses of fluoride caused neurological damage in rats.[5] Fluoride and chlorine have also been shown to interfere with normal thyroid function by inhibiting iodine uptake in the thyroid gland. Since many of the endocrine glands (e.g., the ovaries) normally have high concentrations of iodine, these agents may cause disruptions in the endocrine system.

Dehydration and Autoimmune Disorders. The Common Link: Histamine

As I have discussed in this chapter and as the case studies have supported, water intake has a significant effect on autoimmune disorders. Dr. F. Batmanghelidj writes very eloquently on this subject in his books, <u>Your Body's Many Cries for Water</u> and <u>ABC of Asthma, Allergies and Lupus,</u> two books that I highly recommend.

Histamine is an important neurotransmitter that is produced by the white blood cells throughout the body. It is the primary "water regulating" agent in the body. Histamine acts to shunt water from areas with high water content to areas with low water content. For example, when asthmatics exercise, water is often shunted from the lungs to the muscles of the body, a process that can lead to wheezing.

When a person is in a dehydrated state, histamine levels are elevated throughout the body as the body tries to shunt water to the areas of greatest need. This shunting process can worsen the dehydration in various areas of the body. In Janice's case, she felt the dehydration in her back muscles. Other patients feel it in the joints of their hands (as Carol did) and yet others feel it in the lungs (asthmatics). Dehydration affects people in many different ways.

Elevated histamine levels also present a problem for the immune system. Dr Batmanghelidj claims, "Dehydration that causes the production and release of more than a certain amount of histamine will, in the long run, automatically suppress the immune system of the body -- at its bone marrow site. This is exactly how and why the immune system cannot cope with other diseases, including cancer, when the body has suffered 'drought' for some time."[6] A recent study showed that increased water intake was associated with a reduced risk of colorectal cancer in men. The men who consumed the most water had a 92% lower risk of rectal cancer than those who drank the least water.[7] My experience has shown that in those who suffer with autoimmune disorders, such as rheumatoid arthritis, Lupus and Crohn's, dehydration is often one of their major health issues.

In addition, elevated histamine levels are responsible for producing the signs and symptoms of allergies. It has been known for many years that the inhibition of histamine can improve allergy symptoms and that is the reason that antihistamine medications are so widespread in conventional medicine.

Antihistamine medications have been used to treat a wide range of disorders including the following:

1. Allergies
2. Asthma
3. Peptic Ulcer Disease

163

4. Esophageal Reflux

5. Urticaria (i.e., hives)

6. Dermatitis

In all of the above conditions, antihistamine medications do not treat the underlying reason of why histamine levels are elevated. Antihistamine medications merely block the release of histamine from the cells of the body. As mentioned before, histamine is an important neurotransmitter that regulates water flow in the body. I am convinced that it is not wise to use drugs on a long-term basis to block the important chemical histamine.

When we chemically block the release of histamine from the cells of the body, we are blocking an important messenger molecule (histamine) from performing its many functions, one of which is the regulation of water flow in the body. We should be focusing our energies on causative factors of why histamine levels are elevated in the first place. My experience has shown that histamine levels are often elevated because the body is dehydrated.

The Benefits of Salt

In conventional medical training, doctors are taught the dangers of salt use. In particular, most physicians believe that salt use leads to, and exacerbates, hypertensive states. This line of reasoning, however, does not take into account thousands of years of using salt as a medical tool; and it ignores literature showing the benefits of salt. Furthermore, this line of reasoning ignores common sense.

Salt, like any substance, has good properties and bad properties. When used appropriately, salt is a most important substance for the body; it can help the healing process and it can promote a healthy state. In arthritic conditions salt can act as a medicinal tool to help improve joint mobility. Salt is stored in the cartilage of joints in order to osmotically attract water. This water aids in the lubrication and easy gliding of one joint surface over another.

Salt has the following additional healing properties:

1. It improves allergies by acting as a natural antihistamine.
2. It clears excess acidity from the body.
3. It produces energy in the body.
4. It thins out excess mucous.

However, salt, like all substances can cause problems in the body. When the body is in a dehydrated condition salt can exacerbate a hypertensive problem. Salt acts as an osmotic agent and can worsen a dehydrated condition by pulling more water out of the dehydrated cells. Therefore, when a patient is dehydrated, salt use should be restricted. Also, when in a state of kidney failure, the body may not be able to rid itself of excess salt; in this case, caution must be observed with the use of salt.

Conversely, when the body is in a fully hydrated state, salt has many wonderful uses. Salt, like water, is a natural antihistamine. As I discussed before, when a person is dehydrated, the water-regulating chemical histamine is elevated, leading to or exacerbating problems with immune system disorders (rheumatoid arthritis, Lupus, Crohn's, scleroderma, raynaud's and others). In addition, a salt deficit will worsen other conditions, such as asthma, depression, chronic fatigue and osteoporosis.

I believe that it is wise to utilize the wonderful properties of salt in our diets. Unfortunately, the salt commonly in use today is the wrong kind of salt, and it is harmful to the body. Refined salt is the most common kind of salt in use today. The refining process has removed most of the eighty minerals that are present in unrefined salt. In addition, refined salt has a high content of aluminum that may be associated with many chronic disorders, including Alzheimer's. Unrefined sea salt, on the other hand, contains, in trace amounts, over eighty minerals that our bodies need to perform a wide range of functions. When used in combination with water, sea salt is a wonderful tool to promote healing in the body.

Recommendations: Water

With all of the various sources of water available (from bottled water to tap water) what kind of water do I recommend? I recommend using a water filter that removes fluoride and chlorine, as well as bacteria and parasites. There are many water filters that are worth investigating. An environmental laboratory that specializes in water testing can test your water. Their phone numbers can be found in the Yellow Pages under "water testing." Since a filter system removes many minerals from tap water, as well as the toxic agents mentioned above, it is important that you add a daily multiple vitamin-mineral supplement to your dietary regimen.

My primary recommendation on the use of water is that you ensure an adequate water intake every day. It is impossible to achieve optimum health or to recover from a chronic illness without adequate water intake. I recommend that you take your weight in pounds, divide it by two and use this figure as the amount of water in ounces to ingest on a daily basis. (See Figure 6.) People who are more active will need to further increase their daily intake of water.

---

1. Weight in pounds_____ /2.
2. Result is recommended water intake in ounces
3. Number of ounces _____ /8 = _____ glasses of water per day.

Figure 6: Recommended Water Intake

Recommendations: Salt

Along with my recommendation that you ensure an adequate water intake, I also recommend the use of unrefined sea salt. I suggest starting every day with a pinch of unrefined sea salt, placed on the tongue and followed by a glass of water. I recommend using unrefined sea salt (the Celtic version may be the best form), which can be found in health food stores. In addition, before any heavy exercise, I recommend the use of a pinch of sea salt with a glass of water. Dr. Batmanghelidj recommends a half-teaspoon of sea salt for every ten glasses of water. Again, for further information I refer the reader to Dr. Batmanghelidj's wonderful books, <u>Your Body's Many Cries for Water</u> and <u>ABC of Asthma, Allergies and Lupus</u> and his website www.watercure.com.

[1] Batmanghelidj, F. ABC of Asthma, Allergies and Lupus. Global Health Solutions. 2000.

[2] Family Practice News, vol. 28, no.20. 11/15/98

[3] Sutton, P.R.N. "Is the Ingestion of Fluoride an Immunosuppressive Practice?" Medical Hypothesis, 1991, 35, 1-3.

[4] " Interview of Dr. Yiamouyiannis." Nutrition and Healing, Vol. 4, No. 11. November, 1997

[5] Verner, Julie, et al. "Chronic administration of aluminum-fluoride or sodium-fluoride to rats in drinking water: alterations in neuronal and cerbrovascular integrity." Brain Research, Vol. 784:1998.

[6] Batmanghelidj, F, IBID

[7] International Journal of Cancer 1999; 82:484-489

Chapter 9

Nutritional Supplementation

Nutritional Supplementation

This chapter was written to assist readers in choosing the right supplements to augment their therapies. Choosing supplements can be a daunting task. Health food stores carry hundreds of different brands of supplements. How do you decide which brand of Vitamin C to choose? This chapter will help answer this question and provide the reader with important information on the use of nutritional supplements. This chapter will be organized into five sections:

1. How to choose supplements
2. Why you need to choose supplements
3. Which supplements you should take for arthritis
4. The importance of Niacinamide (Vitamin B-3) in arthritic disorders
5. Why it is important to take the supplements, Glucosamine and Chondroiten Sulfate

How To Choose Supplements

Presently, there is no regulation of supplements by the FDA. As consumers, we are at the mercy of companies to provide exactly what they say is on the label. It is very important for the consumer to compare different products and different manufacturers. My experience has shown that not all supplements are created equal. In fact, not all products are reliable. Some products do not even contain the ingredients that are advertised on the label.

I have found that the quality of some of the over-the-counter supplements is poor. Either they do not contain the amount of the substance that is advertised, or the substance is in a non-absorbable form. For example, many of my patients take DHEA, an adrenal hormone (see Chapter 5), which they have purchased over-the-counter. When I check DHEA levels on these patients, approximately 80% of the time the DHEA levels do not correlate with the dosage on the label of the product. Changing the brand of the DHEA supplement to a more reliable product (i.e., one made by a compounding pharmacist) usually produces the desired result. I have found similar results with other nutritional products, including vitamins, minerals and herbs.

So what do you do? I have found that the best results can be achieved by using products from reliable manufacturers. A reputable manufacturer should be able to provide data on the purity and the content of every batch of the product produced. Furthermore, the products should be made from natural sources, commonly known as whole food sources, and should not contain any dyes, sugars or artificial flavors. Supplements should not be made with harsh detergents, and the ingredients used should be certified organic. In addition, companies should have full control over the buying and processing of the raw ingredients (i.e., they should have in-house processing).

It can be difficult to find a company that meets all of these qualifications; however, there are several good companies that are producing excellent products. The following are some of the companies that I rely on for my products:

1. Biotics Research (800-437-1298)
2. Thorne Research (800-228-1966)
3. Metagenics (800-692-9400)
4. Dragon River Herbs (800-813-2118)
5. Hanna Kreuger Herbs (800-795-0338)
6. Bio Tech Pharmacal, Inc. (800-345-1199)

I recommend that as consumers we all <u>think</u> about which products we are going to use before we purchase them. Using good products can be critical to improving your health and overcoming illness. A knowledgeable health care provider, skilled in the use of nutritional products, can work with you to find the highest quality supplements.

Why Do You Need To Take Supplements?

The best way to obtain adequate amounts of vitamins and minerals is by eating healthy, whole foods. If you eat a healthy diet, why should you supplement it with vitamins and minerals? There are three main reasons that I recommend vitamin and mineral supplements:

1. Poor farming techniques have depleted many soils of vital minerals. Food grown in these depleted soils will contain inadequate mineral levels.

2. Modern food processing has stripped valuable vitamins and minerals from food. Examples of foods that have been stripped of their nutrients include refined flour, refined sugar and partially hydrogenated oils.

3. Fruits and vegetables have been contaminated by the widespread use of pesticides. The antibiotics and hormones given to animals are another source of contamination. These contaminated foods cause oxidative damage in the body.

When we eat food rich in nutrients, the body will use these nutrients to aid in digestion. Eating food that is lacking proper nutrients or that has been contaminated by chemicals, forces our body to use its own store of vitamins and minerals to properly digest the food. This will cause the body to become depleted of these items and may contribute to a poorly functioning immune system.

Vitamins

Vitamins are organic substances found in food that are necessary in small amounts to maintain the body's metabolism and to promote a healthy hormonal system and a strong immune system. There are over fifty vitamins known today. Since vitamins are not manufactured in our bodies, they must be absorbed from our food. They act as co-factors or catalysts for various reactions in the body, and they are best absorbed when in their natural form as whole food components. Those who suffer from a chronic disorder often have depleted levels of some vitamins.

Minerals

Minerals are inorganic substances found in the earth's crust. As with vitamins, minerals are necessary for health and to treat and prevent illness. Minerals, like vitamins, are also depleted in the food supply due to poor farming techniques and food processing. Examples of minerals are calcium, magnesium, zinc and copper. As mentioned above with vitamins, my experience has shown that those with a chronic disorder will often have sub-optimal levels of minerals. It is rare to find a patient suffering from a chronic disorder who does not have some nutritional deficiencies.

A basic multiple vitamin-mineral product is important to use on a daily basis. It provides a wide range of necessary substances, and this variety prevents any single nutrient from becoming depleted. In addition, it may decrease the risk of cancer. A recent study of 88,756 registered nurses showed that the long-term use of a multiple vitamin decreased the risk of colon cancer by 75%.[1]

Maintaining adequate levels of vitamins and minerals in the body is essential to overcoming chronic illness and achieving good health. Those suffering with a chronic illness, such as arthritis, will need a proper nutritional evaluation. This evaluation should include the following tests:

1. Hair analysis for mineral content, including calcium, magnesium, zinc, copper, chromium and selenium levels

2. Serum analysis for magnesium, iron, zinc, Vitamin B12, Folic Acid, Vitamin B6, and Vitamin D levels

In my experience, many of the other nutritional tests that are currently available do not provide consistent results. I believe that taking a good health history (including a diet history), doing a thorough physical exam, and looking at the results of the above tests can provide useful information on the nutritional status of the individual

Recommendations

This section of the book will contain my recommendations for nutritional support of the individual suffering from a chronic illness such as arthritis. Though I will make specific recommendations, the reader must keep in mind that each person has his or her own unique biochemical and nutritional needs.

Fifty years ago, the biochemist Dr. Roger Williams wrote a book on this concept titled, Biochemical Individuality. In 1956, Dr. Williams described the differences in the anatomy and biochemistry in each person.[2] These differences explain why some individuals need higher levels (and some, lower levels) of nutrients than others.

Each person is unique and has a different biochemical make-up. Therefore, when using nutritional supplements, the best results can be achieved by the creation of a unique nutritional program tailored by a health care practitioner to the patient's own biochemical and nutritional needs. I recommend that you work with a health care practitioner who is skilled in the use of natural items and who can work with you to optimize your nutritional status.

Niacinamide

One particular nutrient, niacinamide (Vitamin B-3), is often very effective at reversing symptoms of arthritis. Research done in 1949 showed that niacinamide improved joint mobility and pain in patients with rheumatoid arthritis and osteoarthritis.[3] In 1996, these results were confirmed, and it was further shown that the use of niacinamide allowed the patients to reduce their anti-inflammatory medications.[4]   In a majority of arthritic patients, I have found good results (reduced joint swelling, increased mobility of joints) using niacinamide at doses of 1500-3000mg per day. These doses need to be monitored by a nutritionally oriented health care practitioner.   The following case history can describe the benefits of niacinamide in treating arthritic disorders.

Betty, age 58, had suffered with osteoarthritis for over ten years. "The aching in my joints is intolerable. It is a deep ache, that goes to the core of my joints," she said.   Betty had tried numerous anti-inflammatory medications that provided some relief, but she had side effects to the medications.   Upon taking 1000mg of niacinamide three times per day, along with increasing her water intake, the joint pain began to subside within two weeks. "When I started taking niacinamide, the joint pain began improving immediately.   I could not understand how taking a vitamin could make me feel so good. Recently, I went on a trip for two weeks and forgot to take the niacinamide.   At the end of the trip I started to get the pain and stiffness back.   Now that I am taking it again, the joint pain and stiffness is gone," she claimed.

Supplement Recommendations

The remainder of this section will deal with specific vitamin and mineral recommendations that allow the body to overcome chronic illness and promote healing reactions. Though this list does not cover all vitamins and minerals, it does contain the items that I have found most effective in treating a chronic illness such as arthritis. They include the following:

1. A multiple vitamin-mineral product As previously mentioned, a good multi-vitamin mineral product is essential to providing the body with a rich source of nutrients. Furthermore, it can help keep imbalances from occurring because it contains a wide variety of different vitamins and minerals.

2. Vitamin A Vitamin A is an anti-oxidant. Inadequate levels of this vitamin may lead to hypothyroidism. Vitamin A is found in animal sources. I recommend 10,000 IU per day. Pregnant women may need lower levels.

3. Vitamin B Complex The B vitamins have a wide range of functions in the body, from maintaining the immune system to affecting all of the hormonal glands. B vitamins are commonly stripped from processed food. Inadequate Vitamin B levels will contribute to chronic disease. B vitamins are found in animal products, grains, nuts and seeds. Recommended dose: B-100, two times a day.

4. Vitamin B-3 (Niacinamide): Recommended dose: 1,500-3000mg per day. Please see

Niacinamide section above.

5. Vitamin B-6   Recommended dose: 100mg per day.

6. Vitamin B-12 Vitamin B12 is found only in foods of animal origin, such as dairy, eggs, meat, fish and poultry. It is often deficient in those with a chronic illness. Recommended dose: 1000mg by injection two to three times per week. I recommend only the hydroxycobalamine form of injectable Vitamin B12 and not the cyanocobalamine form of injectable B12.

7. Vitamin C   Vitamin C functions as an important anti-oxidant in the body. Vitamin C is necessary to promote healing and is essential to maintaining joint integrity in the body. Rheumatoid arthritis patients have been shown to have a reduced Vitamin C level in their blood serum. The major dietary sources of Vitamin C are fruits and vegetables. Recommended dose: 3000-5000mg per day.

8. Vitamin D   Vitamin D is necessary for maintaining the structural integrity of bones and teeth. It also is important for maintaining a healthy hormonal system. I have found very low levels of Vitamin D in patients with

arthritis. Vitamin D is found in animal sources, and it can also be made in our bodies by exposure to sunlight. Recommended dose: 1000-2000 Units per day. Vitamin D levels should be checked periodically.

9. Vitamin E Vitamin E and Vitamin C have synergistic effects in the body. Supplementing with Vitamin E has been shown to reduce osteoarthritic symptoms.[5] Vitamin E is found in unrefined vegetable oils, animal products, nuts and leafy green vegetables. Recommended dose: 400-800 I.U. per day of mixed Tocopherols.

Mineral Recommendations

As previously mentioned, adequate mineral levels are necessary to promote health and initiate healing of a chronic illness. For arthritic patients, the most common minerals I recommend supplementing are the following:

1. Magnesium Magnesium is essential for catalyzing hundreds of reactions in the body. A diet high in carbohydrates and processed food can cause a deficiency of magnesium. It is

impossible to maintain health without adequate magnesium levels. Inadequate magnesium levels lead to a poorly functioning immune and hormonal system. Magnesium is found in animal products, nuts and vegetables. Recommended dose: 400mg per day.

2. Calcium   Calcium is essential to maintain the structural integrity of the body; it is a vital component of strong bones and teeth. Inadequate calcium intake is associated with osteoporosis. Drinking large amounts of soda can lead to low calcium levels. In addition, adequate Vitamin D levels are necessary for proper absorption of calcium. Calcium is found in vegetables, nuts, dairy and fish. Recommended dose: 1000-1500mg per day of calcium citrate.

3. Selenium   Selenium acts as an anti-oxidant in the body. It is also important for proper thyroid function. Studies have shown (as has my clinical experience) that low selenium levels are common in arthritic patients.[6]   Selenium is found in nuts, seafood and grains. Recommended dose: 200-400 micrograms per day.

4. Zinc   Zinc has anti-inflammatory effects. Zinc

has been shown to reduce joint swelling, morning stiffness and the subjective assessment of overall disease activity in rheumatoid arthritis.[7] Zinc deficiencies cause problems in the immune system, hormonal system and the prostate gland. Zinc is found in nuts, animal sources and fish. Recommended dose: 25-50mg per day.

5. <u>Copper</u> Copper also has anti-inflammatory effects. If copper levels are low (information gained by a hair analysis) in an arthritic patient, I use small amounts of copper and have observed good results. One study showed benefits in arthritic patients who wore copper bracelets.[8] Recommended dose: 1-4mg per day.

Glucosamine Sulfate and Chondroiten Sulfate

Glucosamine sulfate and chondroiten sulfate are important substances necessary for the body to heal damaged joints (a result of arthritis). These two supplements were popularized in Jason Theodosakis' book, <u>The Arthritis Cure.</u> I have seen good results when arthritic patients supplement with these compounds. Though

I will briefly review these supplements, I refer the reader to Dr. Theodosakis' excellent book.

Glucosamine is an amino acid derivative and is a major building block in the production and maintenance of cartilage in the joints of the body. It also acts to provide structure to the bones, skin, hair, nails and other tissues.

When the joints of the body are damaged, as in arthritis, glucosamine sulfate provides the body with the basic building blocks to begin repairing the damage. Numerous studies have shown that glucosamine sulfate also acts as an anti-inflammatory agent (i.e., a pain reliever).

Chondroiten sulfate is a major component of cartilage. It helps to hold water in the cartilage and acts to facilitate the transfer of nutrients into the cartilage. It has been shown to improve joint destruction in those who suffer with osteoarthritis.[9] It is derived from the cartilage of animals.

The literature is clear on the benefits of using both glucosamine sulfate and chondroiten sulfate in the treatment of osteoarthritic joints. Both of these agents stimulate the production of new cartilage in injured joints of the body. In addition, these supplements have synergistic effects with one another; in other words, they work better together than they do when used separately.

In comparing glucosamine sulfate and chondroiten sulfate with the more commonly used NSAID's (i.e., nonsteroidal anti-inflammatory drugs such as aspirin or Motrin), one must keep in mind that glucosamine and chondroiten sulfate not only have anti-inflammatory effects in the joints, but they also promote the healing of these areas. NSAIDS, on the other hand, have never been shown to promote healing, and the long-term use of these agents has been shown to actually inhibit healing in the joints of the body. It is clear that glucosamine sulfate and chondroiten sulfate, instead of NSAIDS, should be the first line of treatment for any form of arthritis.

Recommended Doses of Glucosamine Sulfate and Chondroiten Sulfate

For arthritic conditions I recommend the following doses: glucosamine sulfate- 500 mg three times per day and chondroiten sulfate- 400mg three times per day. These supplements work best when used in combination, rather than individually.

Herbs

Herbs have been used in many different cultures to help control the symptoms of arthritis. Ginger has been used as a natural anti-inflammatory agent for thousands of years. One to two grams per day of ginger has proven effective in relieving many of the symptoms of arthritis. Research has also shown the herb feverfew to be effective in improving the symptoms of arthritis.[10]

Final Thoughts

Nutritional supplements are important elements that provide the body with essential nutrients to promote healing of injured areas. They also provide the basic building blocks to promote the health of the individual.

As previously mentioned, due to our poor food supply, it is nearly impossible to obtain from our diet all of the nutrients we need to maintain health. I encourage readers to do their own research about which supplements might be beneficial to their health. Work with a knowledgeable health care provider who has experience with natural supplements. If your health care provider does not share your views about using natural items, I suggest you find one who is in agreement with your views. Any treatment modality can be improved with a sound nutritional approach that supplies your body with the basic building blocks to promote healing and good health.

[1] "Family Practice News." December 1, 1998, p. 31.

[2] Williams, Roger. Biochemical Individuality. Keats. 1956

[3] Kaufman, W. The common form of Joint Dysfunction: Its Incidence and Treatment. E.L. Hildreth Co., Brattleboro, Vt. 1949

[4] Jonas, W.B., et al. "The effect of niacinamide on osteoarthritis: a pilot study." Inflamm. Res. 1996;45:330-334

[5] Machtey, I., eta l. " Tocopherol in osteoarthritis: a controlled pilot study." J. Am. Ger. Soc. 1978; 26:328-330.

[6] Tarp, U., et al. " Low selenium level in severe rheumatoid arthritis." Scand. J. Rheum. 1985; 14:97

[7] Simkin, PA. " Oral zinc sulphate in rheumatoid arthritis." Lancet. 1976;2:539-542

[8] Walker, WR. Et al. " An investigation of the therapeutic value of the 'copper bracelet:' dermal assimilation f copper in arthritic/rheumatoid conditions." Agents Actions 1976; 6:454-459

[9] Kerzberg, EM, et al. "Combination of glycosaminoglycans and acetylsalicylic acid in knee osteoarthritis.: Scand. J. Rheum. 1987; 16:377

[10] Heptinstall, Patrick, M. " Feverfew in rheumatoid arthritis: a double blind, placebo-controlled study. " Ann. Rheum Dis. 1989;48;547

Chapter 10

Detoxification

Detoxification

This chapter will explain how exposure to chemicals can affect our bodies and how important it is to "detoxify" our bodies from the various chemicals and toxins that poison the cells. Exposure to harmful chemicals and toxins can adversely affect our immune system, which can further lead to poor health and chronic illness. It has been my experience that many of those who suffer from chronic illness often have high levels of toxic elements in their bodies. When these toxic items are removed, through a detoxification plan, the patient's health will begin to improve. This chapter will show you how to identify which items may be toxic and how to remove them.

We are exposed to a variety of chemicals (from common household cleaners to pesticides to food additives) every day. Our body has to process all of these chemicals and remove harmful substances from our system. The removal of harmful substances from our body is a two-stage process that begins in the liver. First the chemical substance is rendered harmless in the liver, and then the chemical substance is removed from the body by one of three ways: sweating, stool or urination.

Problems develop when our detoxification pathways become overwhelmed as a result of overexposure to harmful chemicals. When the detoxification pathways become overwhelmed, the liver is unable to remove these substances; and the body has no place to store them. These dangerous substances then begin to accumulate in different cells of the body. This accumulation of harmful substances can result in the cells of the body becoming poisoned. As more and more cells of the body lose their ability to work properly, the immune system will start to malfunction. The immune system will no longer be able to ward off invading organisms and the body will therefore become more susceptible to illness.

When the immune system becomes unable to control various infectious agents such as bacteria, viruses and parasites, the stage is set for chronic illnesses to develop. The resulting problems can include arthritis, fibromyalgia, cancer, autoimmune disorders, fatigue and allergies. I have found it nearly impossible to treat a chronic illness without adequately addressing toxicity in the body.

As previously stated, the liver is the major detoxifying organ in the body. The liver is the largest organ in the body and is located in the upper right abdomen, behind the rib cage. In addition to detoxification, the liver has many other functions including the following:

1. Storing vitamins and minerals such as Vitamin A, Vitamin B-12, Vitamin D, copper, iron, etc.
2. Regulating carbohydrate metabolism
3. Controlling protein metabolism
4. Facilitating fat absorption

It is vitally important to maintain a healthy liver because it has such a wide range of essential functions in the body. A healthy liver is maintained by eating a diet free of pesticides, synthetic hormones and other toxins. In addition, eliminating refined foods, especially refined sugar and flour, helps to promote a healthy liver.

When the liver is not functioning appropriately, it is impossible to achieve optimum health. Often those who suffer with a chronic illness, such as arthritis, will have a poorly functioning liver. In order to overcome illness, a proper liver detoxification program must be undertaken: the liver must be cleansed so that it may perform all of the above functions.

The liver detoxifies toxic substances by making them water-soluble and allowing the kidneys to release them through the urine. Those substances not released in the urine are released in the stool.

Heavy metals are a major cause of toxicity in the liver. Heavy metal toxicity occurs when an individual has been exposed to a heavy metal, and this toxin becomes absorbed into his or her system. Heavy metals can wreak havoc with one's immune and hormonal systems. Heavy metals include the following:

1. Mercury
2. Lead
3. Arsenic
4. Cadmium
5. Nickel
6. Aluminum

I have found heavy metal toxicity in a large number of patients suffering from a chronic illness. Is heavy metal toxicity the cause of the chronic illness in these individuals or just one of several factors inhibiting the normal function of their immune system? I believe that most chronic illness is a result of a number of factors, one being heavy metal toxicity. A proper detoxification program is necessary to cleanse the liver and to help the body overcome a chronic illness.

This chapter will describe the six heavy metals listed above and show you why these items are toxic to the body. At the end of the chapter I will review specific detoxification procedures that I have found helpful in removing these toxic substances.

Mercury

The U.S. Department of Health and Human Services lists

mercury as the third most hazardous substance known to mankind.[1] The World Health Organization states that there is no minimum level of mercury that does not cause harm. The number one source of mercury poisoning is dental fillings. Dental amalgams (i.e., fillings) contain approximately 50% mercury as well as other metals, including nickel. The World Health Organization estimates that the largest source of mercury in humans comes from fillings implanted by dentists. The amount of mercury from fillings is over ten times more than for all other environmental sources combined.[2]

Mercury is also found in sources other than dental fillings. The following are some of the other sources of mercury:

1. Fish
2. Water-based paint
3. Polluted water
4. Fungicides
5. Some pesticides
6. Immunizations
7. Some cosmetics
8. Soft contact lens solutions

The American Academy of Pediatrics and the U.S. Public Health Service recently asked vaccine manufacturers to remove mercury from their vaccines. Mercury was put in the vaccines to act as a preservative. I believe that children should not be given immunizations with mercury in them.

A study recently released estimates that each year in the United States 60,000 children are born with neurological problems resulting from exposure to mercury. Newborns can acquire mercury toxicity from their mother.[3]

Mercury is a known cell toxin that can cause imbalances in the immune system and can interfere with normal hormonal function. The thyroid gland and the pituitary/hypothalamic glands are very sensitive to mercury. Mercury is easily absorbed from the fillings in the mouth. It can be released as a vapor in the mouth, and chewing exacerbates its release. In fact, studies have shown that gum chewing can increase the release of mercury in the form of mercury vapor by 1,560%. Once released, mercury is easily absorbed in the body and concentrates in numerous tissues, including the following:

1. Brain
2. Kidney
3. Gastrointestinal tract
4. Liver
5. Fetal tissue (from the mother's fillings)[4]

Mercury is toxic to the body's own genetic material (DNA). Researchers have found a significant correlation between the amount of mercury in the body and the number of DNA aberrations.[5] In addition, mercury blocks enzyme functions throughout the body and decreases protein synthesis. Mercury exposure from dental fillings has also been linked to Alzheimer's disease and Amyotrophic Lateral Sclerosis (ALS) by researchers at the University of Kentucky.[6]

Studies have shown higher mercury concentrations in the brain and kidneys of individuals who have mercury fillings versus those who do not have mercury fillings. Research has also shown a correlation with the number of fillings and the amount of mercury in the body. In addition, studies with animals have shown that mercury fillings can induce autoimmune diseases.

I cannot fathom why dentists still use mercury fillings when the danger and toxicity of mercury is a well-known fact. It is my opinion that mercury amalgams should be banned, as has been done in some European countries. If you suffer from a chronic disease such as arthritis, chronic fatigue syndrome or fibromyalgia, you may want to have your mercury fillings replaced with non-mercury fillings.

Often, the removal of mercury fillings can be done gradually, as the fillings need to be replaced. However, the presence of a chronic illness will often necessitate a more urgent response. Whether you should have your mercury fillings removed should be discussed with a health care provider who is knowledgeable about mercury toxicity.

Remove The Source

The first rule of toxicology is to remove the source of the problem. One of the major sources of mercury is dental amalgams. Does everyone who has mercury fillings need to have their fillings replaced with non-mercury fillings? There is no clear-cut answer. I do not advocate the immediate removal of mercury fillings unless there is a medical reason. As previously mentioned, I would recommend mercury amalgam removal for those who suffer with a chronic illness, such as an autoimmune disorder or cancer. For those people who are in good health, the answer is not as clear.

I recommend that you work with a dentist knowledgeable about the toxic effects of mercury and skilled in the proper procedure for removing mercury fillings. The incorrect removal of mercury fillings can actually result in higher mercury levels being released in the body. In addition, I recommend that you work with a health care practitioner who is knowledgeable about mercury toxicity and skilled in the use of agents to detoxify the body. Mercury is a very dangerous substance; often it takes a "team" working together to get the best results. The removal of mercury fillings is an expensive process and one that must be done with great care. A dentist who is knowledgeable about the dangers of mercury can be found by contacting the following organizations:

1. DAMS organization: (800) 311-6265

2. International Academy of Oral Medical Toxicology (IAOMT): (407) 299-4149

My experience has shown that elevated mercury levels are directly correlated with chronic illnesses such as arthritis, fibromyalgia, autoimmune disorders, cancer and others. I have consistently seen higher mercury levels in those who suffer from a chronic illness. A question to ponder is this: "Is mercury the causative factor in these illnesses, or is it one of many other factors?" I am not sure of the answer, but I have seen very positive results when mercury is removed and mercury levels are lowered.

Mercury levels can be assessed through hair and urine testing. I have found two substances extremely useful for chelating (i.e., binding) the mercury in the body and allowing its excretion through the urine or stool: DMPS (2,3-Dimercapto-1-Propanesulfolic Acid) and DMSA (2,3- Dimercaptosuccinic Acid). I have found these agents extremely helpful in diagnosing and treating elevated mercury levels. For more information on the uses of DMPS and DMSA, please see the sections "Testing for Heavy Metal Toxicity" and "Treating Heavy Metal Toxicity."

Lead

Lead is an environmental pollutant that is very toxic to humans. In young children, it acts as a neurotoxin and can adversely affect intelligence, concentration and language development. Lead toxicity can lead to ADHD, headaches, fatigue, muscle pains, indigestion, tremors, constipation and poor coordination. Lead is also a potent enzyme inhibitor in the body. Sources of lead include air pollution, bone meal supplements, water that has passed through lead pipes, batteries, lead paint, cigarette smoke and hair dyes.

Arsenic

Arsenic is an environmental pollutant. Arsenic, at high levels, can cause many neurotoxic effects, including headaches, drowsiness, confusion, weakness and skin problems. It has been associated with anemia, kidney and liver problems, hypertension, heart failure and skin cancers. Sources of arsenic include industrial pollution, insecticides, seafood and auto exhaust. It can also be released into wells and ground water from underground mineral sources.

Cadmium

Cadmium is an industrial pollutant. Cadmium toxicity can cause high blood pressure, anemia and kidney and liver damage. It can also impair calcium absorption and influence the development of osteoporosis. Sources of cadmium include industrial waste, auto exhaust and cigarette smoke. It can also be found in some refined foods (especially white flour and rice), fertilizers, batteries and sewage sludge.

Nickel

Nickel is a heavy metal that is toxic at high levels but does have an essential role in the body at low levels. At low levels, nickel may help stabilize the building blocks of our bodies, the DNA and the RNA. In addition, small amounts of nickel have been used to successfully treat psoriasis.

Nickel can be ingested, inhaled or absorbed through the skin. Sources of nickel include tobacco smoke, dental fillings, dental appliances, industrial pollution, batteries, hydrogenated fats, fertilizers and acidic food cooked in stainless steel cookware. Also, the manufacturing process for margarine and shortening requires the use of nickel. It is impossible to remove all traces of nickel from margarine and shortening.

Aluminum

Aluminum toxicity is widespread in this country. Aluminum toxicity has been linked to neurological disorders, including Alzheimer's and Parkinson's disorder. Poor memory, confusion, depression, learning disorders and hyperactivity have been associated with aluminum toxicity.

Aluminum is found in a wide range of consumer products:

baking powder, anti-perspirants, processed cheese, antacids, table salt (processed with aluminum), aluminum pots and pans, cigarettes, aluminum foil, pesticides, artificial coloring and aluminum-treated white flour. It is best to keep aluminum exposure to a minimum by avoiding the products listed above.

Testing for Heavy Metal Toxicity

It is imperative that those who suffer with a chronic illness be appropriately evaluated and treated for heavy metal toxicity. I have found elevated heavy metal levels (especially mercury) in a large number of my patients who suffer from a chronic illness, such as arthritis, chronic fatigue, autoimmune disorders and cancer.

Heavy metal toxicity can set the stage for a chronic illness to appear, or it may be one of many items contributing to disease and poor health. In either case, the removal of heavy metals, through a proper detoxification program, can help the immune system function at a higher level.

An evaluation of heavy metals may begin first with a hair evaluation. Hair testing has been shown to be a reliable indicator of the body's level of heavy metals. Hair testing is inexpensive and can provide additional information on the mineral status of the body. Hair testing, however, should not be the only method used to diagnose heavy metal toxicities.

Urine challenge testing has also proven to be a very reliable way to test for heavy metal toxicity. I have found urine challenge testing to be more sensitive and more specific than hair testing. Therefore, in those who suffer from a chronic illness, I believe a urine challenge test should be utilized to properly evaluate for heavy metal toxicity.

A urine challenge test is performed by taking a chelating (i.e., binding) agent. The most common substances used are DMPS and DMSA. These agents have a high affinity for binding to many heavy metals in the body. After the metals are bound by the DMPS or the DMSA, they will be excreted in the urine or the stool. (See the box below.)

Heavy Metal Challenge Test

1. Ensure adequate kidney function.
2. Check 24-hour urine for heavy metals.
3. Take a chelating agent (DMPS or DMSA).
4. Collect 24-hour urine output.
5. Check the urine for heavy metals.

DMPS is given by injection (3mg/kg of body weight). DMSA is given orally, usually in a single 500 mg dose. After taking either agent, urine is collected for six to twenty-four hours and sent to a lab for evaluation.

Case Study

Jessica, age 37, was diagnosed with fibromyalgia at the age of 33 after becoming ill with a flu virus. She reported having most of the symptoms of fibromyalgia, including aching muscles, fatigue, and having a difficult time sleeping. "My life is miserable. I ache all over and I never feel rested. I feel like I have aged twenty years since I became ill," she said. My examination of Jessica revealed hypothyroid and hypoadrenal states. After being treated with appropriate hormonal and nutritional supplementation, Jessica made little improvement. When she was screened with a hair analysis for heavy metals, high levels of mercury were found. The elevated mercury level was later confirmed with a DMPS urine test. Jessica was subsequently treated with DMSA, vitamins and minerals (selenium, Vitamin C, N-acetyl-cysteine, Vitamin E and others) and herbs (cilantro). Three months later, after carefully following her declining mercury levels, she made a dramatic improvement in her health. "It was like a light switch had been turned on. I feel like I have been given my life back. My energy is back to normal and my achiness is gone," she happily reported. Jessica eventually had her mercury fillings taken out and enjoys good health today.

Treating Heavy Metal Toxicity

Once a diagnosis of elevated heavy metals is made, an appropriate detoxification program should be implemented. Detoxification is necessary to allow the immune system to regain strength and to restore the proper functioning of the cells of the body.

A proper detoxification program should contain five steps:

1. Removal of the source of toxicity
2. Improvement of the diet in order to nourish the body
3. Use of the proper medication and nutritional supplements to aid the detoxification pathways
4. Consumption of adequate amounts of water
5. Sweating

Step 1: Remove The Source of Toxicity

As previously mentioned, the first rule of toxicology is to remove the source of the toxic agent(s). When a diagnosis of mercury toxicity is made, all mercury-containing fillings should be removed before instituting a detoxification program.

However, caution must be observed when removing mercury fillings. If proper procedures for removing mercury fillings are not observed, there is a risk of actually increasing the release of mercury vapors in the body.

Proper removal of mercury fillings should be done with a rubber dam, and be performed by a dentist skilled in the proper removal of mercury fillings. Precautions should be taken to minimize the risk of mercury exposure to both the patient and the dentist.

After the mercury fillings have been removed, a challenge test should be performed to see how much mercury is still left in the body. DMSA and DMPS are examples of agents that have been shown to be reliable in testing for mercury (and other heavy metals) levels. The challenge test was described on Page 205.

Step 2: Improve The Diet

The second step in a detoxification program is eating healthy foods that provide vitamins and minerals that aid the body in the detoxification process. I refer the reader to Chapter 6, which provides information on how to properly balance the diet with adequate amounts of protein, fat and carbohydrates.

In order to detoxify your body, it is necessary to reduce (or better yet, eliminate) refined sugar from the diet. Refined sugar contains no nutrients and when eaten in excess will lead to excess obesity and liver dysfunction. Further, I recommend eliminating any intake of artificial sweeteners, including aspartame-containing products, as they are toxic to the liver. Natural sweeteners such as stevia or honey are acceptable.

Eating organic food is very helpful in any detoxification

program. Pesticides on fruits and vegetables (also found in many juices) are extremely toxic to the liver and the fat cells of the body. Organic fruits and vegetables should not contain any pesticide residue.

Hormones contained in most conventional meat products have disastrous effects on the body. Not only are they an added substance the liver has to detoxify, but also many of these hormones, I believe, add to the incidence of cancer, particularly breast and prostate cancer. These hormones also wreak havoc with our own hormonal systems. Therefore, I recommend that you eat meat from organically raised animals only.

In addition, organically raised animals have a more favorable fatty acid profile than do conventionally raised animals. In other words, it is healthier to ingest meat from an organically raised animal, rather than meat from a conventionally raised animal. For a healthier lifestyle, I recommend eating only hormone-free meat products.

Step 3: Taking the Proper Medicine and Nutritional Supplements

It is essential to use nutritional agents that help clear the body's detoxification pathways. I have found that using DMSA (an oral mercury chelating agent) about one hour before removal of mercury fillings can be very helpful in keeping mercury levels low. In addition, the use of supplements can help keep detoxification pathways optimally functioning and help the body rid itself of toxins such as mercury. For a list of supplements recommended, see Figure 7 below.

---

1. Vitamin C: 3000mg/day
2. Vitamin E: 800IU/day
3. Garlic: 500mg/day
4. Cilantro drops: 4/day
5. L-Glutamine: 3-6g/day
6. Selenium: 400mcg/day
7. Multiple vitamin-mineral complex

Figure 7: Nutritional Supplements Recommended for Detoxification

---

Step 4: Drinking Adequate Amounts of Water

It is impossible to properly detoxify the body without adequately hydrating the body. Water helps flush out toxins throughout the body, including from the liver and the kidneys. Also, water can help carry nutrients into the cells.

It is best to drink most of the water between meals, rather than at the meals. To calculate how much water you should ingest, see Figure 8 on the next page.

Water should be the beverage of choice. All sodas should be eliminated. Herbal tea is an accepted beverage, but it is not a substitute for water. Finally, adding a pinch of Celtic Sea Salt per day to the regimen seems to improve the body's utilization of water. (See Chapter 8 for more information.)

Weight in pounds_____/2.
Result is recommended water intake in ounces.
Number of ounces _____/8 = _____ glasses of water per day.

Figure 8: Recommended Water Intake

Step 5: Sweating

Sweating is an important physiologic reaction in the body. Sweating allows the body to rid itself of toxic chemicals and clear the lymph system. Many individuals who suffer from chronic illnesses report that they do not sweat. I recommend using a sauna to help train the body to sweat. I have observed very good results with infra-red saunas.

Final Thoughts

I have included this section on detoxification because detoxifying the body is very important in overcoming chronic illness. In addition, it is nearly impossible to achieve optimal health without a well-functioning liver. I recommend working with a health care provider who is knowledgeable about the problems with heavy metal toxicity and about proper detoxification techniques. A good resource on diet recommendations for maintaining a healthy liver while undergoing a detoxification process can be found in the book, The Liver Cleansing Diet, by Sandra Cabot, M.D.

[1] "ATSDR/EPA Priority List." Agency for Toxic Substances and Disease Registry. US Department of Health and Human Services, 1995

[2] Kennedy, David. Health Consciousness, 1992;13(3);92-93.

[3] Oakland Press, 7/12/2000, A-5

[4] Drasch, G., et al. "Mercury Burden of Human Fetal and Infant Tissues." European Journal of Pediatrics. 1994; 153:607.

[5] Verschaeve, L., et al. "Genetic Damage Induced by Occupationally low Mercury Exposure." Environmental Research. 12:306

[6] Hailey, Boyd. "A Study of the Toxic Effects of Oral Mercury and Bacterial Metabolites Produced in Periodontal Disease and Infected Teeth: Possible Relationship to Alzheimer's Disease." Presented at ACAM, 1999-2000.

Chapter 11

Final Thoughts

Final Thoughts

Now that you have read this book and have begun to see how it is possible to overcome arthritis, fibromyalgia and chronic fatigue syndrome, you may be asking yourself two questions:

1. Where do I start?
2. How do I find a doctor to work with me?

This chapter will give the reader information on how to put together all of the data in this book and how to regain and maintain your health. Often times, taking the first step is the most difficult part of this process.

The first step to achieving your optimal health is to gather knowledge about how you can use safe, natural treatments that promote healing in the body. You have already taken the first step by reading this book. You can now see that it is possible to

217

overcome a chronic illness and achieve optimum health. Now you must use this knowledge and develop a course of action. Take the information that your health care practitioner gives you, do your own research, and come to your own conclusions about how you want to proceed. This book was written to provide you with information on safe and natural items that I have found successful in treating arthritis. You now have the information to make your own health care decisions. An active, informed patient, who takes charge of his or her own medical decisions, will have a better outcome than a passive patient.

The next step to regaining your health includes eating a healthy diet. Dr. Barry Sears, the author of the <u>Zone Books</u> states that, "Food is the most powerful drug we will encounter every day."[1] We must think about the food we eat and eat healthy food that will replenish our bodies with vitamins, minerals, enzymes and other healthy items. Eating a poor diet will ensure failure in overcoming a chronic illness. The Standard American Diet, which includes too many carbohydrates (particularly high glycemic, refined carbohydrates), does not provide enough nutrition to support the immune system. Simply eliminating refined sugar and flour as well as trans fatty acids from the diet is a great place to begin. Once you eliminate these items from your diet, you will begin to see an improvement in your condition. For more information on eating a healthy diet, refer back to Chapter 6.

In addition to changing your diet, it is essential to drink an adequate amount of water. The concept of keeping the body hydrated cannot be overstated, particularly in those that suffer with a chronic illness. I often tell my patients: "Don't bother taking vitamins, minerals, herbs, natural hormones, etc., if you are not going to drink adequate amounts of water. You are wasting your time and money." It sounds too good to be true; simply drinking more water and eliminating other drinks that can lead to dehydration, is a simple and effective way of beginning the healing process.

Determining whether there is an infectious etiology (or cause) of a chronic illness (as described in Chapter 2) is the next step. Unfortunately, conventional medicine, with its reliance on toxic drug therapies that only treat the symptoms of an illness, does not address the underlying cause of the illness. I believe treating the underlying cause of the illness (e.g., infection, nutritional depletion, dehydration, etc.), is the key to overcoming the illness. I have seen countless patients who have been unable to effectively treat arthritis, fibromyalgia, chronic fatigue syndrome and other chronic disorders with drug therapies. Many times these patients will have a dramatic improvement in their condition once an infection is properly treated along with following the holistic parameters outlined in this book.

Using a holistic approach to overcome a chronic illness will ensure a well-functioning immune system. This approach includes ensuring that there are adequate levels of basic nutrients (vitamins, minerals, herbs, natural hormones, etc.), which are necessary to heal injured tissues. For more information on nutritional supplementation, see Chapter 9. Detoxification of the body can also improve the body's utilization of basic nutrients, as explained in Chapter 10.

Having a health care provider that is willing to work with you is an important step. If your provider is unwilling to work with you in devising a holistic approach for you, I suggest finding someone else. Many doctors are reluctant to use natural items because they are not trained in their use. However, as doctors see the positive benefits of using these safe, natural items, they will begin to understand their significance. There are many doctors who do understand the benefits of using natural items and attend conferences to learn more about these items. Two resources that can help you find a health care practitioner knowledgeable about the use of natural items include the following:

1. Broda O. Barnes M.D. Research Foundation, Inc.
   P.O. Box 98
   Trumball, CT 06611
   (203) 261-2101
   The Barnes Foundation specializes in the use of natural hormones and thyroid disorders.

2. American College for the Advancement in Medicine (ACAM)
   23121 Verdugo Drive
   Suite 204
   Laguna Hills, CA 92653
   (800) 532-3688
   ACAM is a medical society that educates physicians in preventive/nutritional medicine.

Sometimes it takes a "team" approach to helping one overcome chronic illness. At my office, we have a nutritionist, hands-on healers, a massage therapist and others. I also utilize chiropractors, compounding pharmacists and many other healing practitioners. Using a team approach to treating a chronic problem is very useful. Your doctor can help you coordinate this.

I cannot overemphasize the importance of maintaining a healthy immune system. Eating a healthy diet, drinking adequate amounts of water and using natural items can be a start to obtaining a healthy immune system. Using drug therapies alone will not promote a healthy immune system.

The steps outlined in the chapters of this book have proven successful in my patients. I believe that following these steps can help you achieve your optimum health and overcome chronic illness. Don't suffer with your illness. Take charge and help your body overcome disease. Remember it is up to you to take an active role in your health care decisions. Using the unique holistic treatments outlined in this book can help you achieve your optimum health.

To all of our health!

[1] Sears, Barry. <u>Enter the Zone.</u> Regan Books. 1995

Appendix A: Glycemic Index of Carbohydrates

The glycemic index is a measure of the speed of entry of carbohydrates into the bloodstream. Since carbohydrates cause blood sugar to rise, resulting in an elevated insulin level, it is recommended to limit the foods with the highest glycemic index and to eat foods with the lowest glycemic index (i.e. those with an index <50%).

High glycemic index, greater than 100% ('Bad' carbohydrates)
Grain-Based Foods
> Puffed rice
> Corn flakes
> Puffed wheat
> Millet
> Instant rice
> Instant potato
> Microwave Potato
> French bread

Simple Sugars
> Maltose
> Glucose

Snacks
> Tofu ice cream
> Puffed-rice cakes

Glycemic Index Standard = 100%
> White Bread

Glycemic Index between 80 and 100%
Grain-based foods
> Grapenuts
> Whole wheat bread
> Rolled oats
> Oat bran
> Instant mashed potatoes

White rice
Brown rice
Muesli
Shredded wheat
Vegetables
Carrots
Parsnips
Corn
Fruits
Banana
Raisins
Apricots
Papaya
Mango
Snacks
Ice cream (low fat)
Corn chips
Rye crisps

Glycemic index between 50 and 80%
Grain-based foods
Spaghetti (white)
Spaghetti (whole wheat)
Pasta, other
Pumpernickel bread
All-bran cereal
Fruits
Orange
Orange juice
Vegetables
Peas
Pinto beans
Garbanzo beans
Kidney beans (canned)
Baked beans
Navy beans
Simple sugars
Lactose
Sucrose

Glycemic index between 30 and 50%
Grain based foods

Barley
Oatmeal (slow cooking)
Whole grain bread
Fruits
Apple
Apple juice
Applesauce
Pears
Grapes
Peaches
Vegetables
Kidney Beans (fresh)
Lentils
Black-eyed peas
Chick-peas
Lima beans
Tomato soup
Peas
Dairy Products
Ice cream (high fat)
Milk
Yogurt

Glycemic index less than 30% ('Good' carbohydrates)

Fruits
Cherries
Plums
Grapefruit
Simple sugars
Fructose
Vegetables
Soy beans
Nuts
Peanuts and other nuts

Appendix B: Resources

How To Find A Doctor Who Is Knowledgeable About Natural Hormones

It can be a daunting task to find a health care practitioner to work with you on using a holistic approach to treat arthritis, fibromyalgia, chronic fatigue syndrome and other chronic illnesses. The following resources are available to you to find a practitioner in your area. It may take trial and error to find a doctor who can work with you. Don't give up if you find it a difficult task. Many times it is a trial and error process to find the right practitioner(s) for you.

Societies That Teach Doctors How To Use Natural Hormones:

1. Broda O. Barnes, M.D., Research Foundation
    P.O. Box 98
    Trumbull, CT 06611
    1-203-261-2101
    Website: www.brodabarnes.org

2. American College for Advancement In Medicine
    23121 Verdugo Dr.
    Suite 204
    Laguna Hills, CA 92653
    1-800-532-3688
    Website: www.acam.org

Information On The Use Of Antibiotics To Treat Arthritis:

The Road Back Foundation
Box 447
Orleans, MA 02653
Website: www.roadback.org

Information On How To Find A Compounding Pharmacist:

International Academy of Compounding Pharmacies (IACP)
P.O. Box 1365
Sugar Land Texas, 77847
1-800-927-4227
Website: www.compassnet.com/iacp

Appendix C: Recommended Reading List

ABC of Asthma, Allergies & Lupus, F. Batmanghelidj, M.D. (Global Health Solutions, Inc. 2000).

The Arthritis Breakthrough, Henry Scammell (M. Evans & Company, Inc., 1993)

The Arthritis Cure, Jason Theodosakis, M.D., Brenda Adderly, M.H.A. & Barry Fox, Ph.D. (St. Martin's Paperbacks, 1997)

Hypothyroidism: The Unsuspected Illness, Broda O. Barnes, M.D. and Lawrence Galton (Harper & Row Publishers, 1976).

The Liver Cleansing Diet, Sandra Cabot, M.D. (S.C.B. International, 1997)

Living Well With Hypothyroidism, Mary J. Shomon (Avon Books, Inc., 2000)

Maximize Your Vitality & Potency, Jonathan Wright, M.D. and Lane Lenard, Ph.D. (Smart Publications, 1999)

The Miracle of Natural Hormones, David Brownstein, M.D. (Medical Alternatives Press, Inc. 1999)

Natural Hormone Replacement For Women Over 45, Jonathan Wright, M.D. and John Morgenthaler. (Smart Publications, 1997)

Safe Uses of Cortisol, William McK. Jefferies, M.D. (Charles C. Thomas Publisher, Ltd. 1996).

Say Goodbye To Illness, Devi S. Nambudripad, D.C. (Delta Publishing Co., 1999)

Your Body's Many Cries for Water, F. Batmanghelidj, M.D. (Smart Publications, 1997)

Index

A

adrenal glands, 33, 40, 41, 43, 47, 69, 71, 73, 91, 92, 94, 95, 96
allergies, 62, 139-149
aluminim.203-204
Armour thyroid,71,73-74,81-82
arsenic, 61,202
autoimmune disorders, 22-24

B

bacterial infection,13-15, 23-28,36-42
basal body temperature,79-80

C

cadmium, 202-203
calcium, 177-178,184
carbohydrates, 129-135
cats claw,16,26
chondroiten sulfate,173,185-187
chronic fatigue syndrome,25, 47-63
copper, 185

D

dehydration 153-164,166-168
detoxification,
DHEA, 87-94
DMPS,205,
DMSA,205

E

enzymes, 122
essential fatty acids,126-129
estradiol, 61, 63
estrogens, 3, 54, 64, 65

F

fat, 123-129
fibromyalgia, 25-,27-28,47-63
flouride,161-162

G

Ginger, 187-188
Glucosamine sulfate, 173,185-187
glycemic index , 223-225 Appendix A

H

Herxheimer reactions, 31-32, 34-35
histamine, 148, 162-164
human growth hormone, 108-113
hydrocortisone, 104-108
hydrogenated oil, 127-129, 176
hypothyroidism, 71-82

I

intravenous antibiotics,32-35

L

lead, 61, 201-202
licorice root,16
lupus, 23,72-73,101-102

M

magnesium, 177-178,183-184
mycoplasma 14-20,24-27,31-33, 36-43
mercury, 61, 196-201

N

niacinamide, 179-182
nickel, 203
NSAIDs, 4, 37-39

P

PCR testing, 41
progesterone, 100-103
protein, 121-123
psoriatic arthritis, 19-20, 22-24

R

rheumatoid arthritis, 16-19, 22-24, 29-31,73-74,133-134

S

salt, 164-166, 168
scleroderma, 22-24, 105-107,
selenium, 184
synthetic hormones, 68-70

T

testosterone, 94-100
thyroid gland, 70-82
trans fatty acids, 128-129
TSH test, 76-78

V

Vasculitis, 21-24, 110-111
Vitamin A, 181
Vitamin B-6, 182
Vitamin B-12, 182
Vitamin C, 182
Vitamin D, 182-183
Vitamin E, 183

W,X,Y,Z

Water, 153-164, 166-167
Zinc, 185

Books by David Brownstein, M.D.
(For more information: www.drbrownstein.com)

IODINE: WHY YOU NEED IT, WHY YOU CAN'T LIVE WITHOUT IT, 3rd EDITION

Iodine is the most misunderstood nutrient. Dr. Brownstein shows you the benefit of supplementing with iodine. Iodine deficiency is rampant. Iodine deficiency is a world-wide problem and is at near epidemic levels in the United States. Most people wrongly assume that you get enough iodine from iodized salt. Dr. Brownstein convincingly shows you why it is vitally important to get your iodine levels measured. He shows you how iodine deficiency is related to:

- Breast cancer
- Hypothyroidism and Graves' disease
- Autoimmune illnesses
- Chronic Fatigue and Fibromyalgia
- Cancer of the prostate, ovaries and much more!

OVERCOMING THYROID DISORDERS 2nd Edition

This book provides new insight into why thyroid disorders are frequently undiagnosed and how best to treat them. The holistic treatment plan outlined in this book will show you how safe and natural remedies can help improve your thyroid function and help you achieve your optimal health.

- Detoxification
- Diet
- Graves'
- Hashimoto's Disease
- Hypothyroidism
- And Much More!!

DRUGS THAT DON'T WORK and NATURAL THERAPIES THAT DO

This book will show you why the most commonly prescribed drugs may not be your best choice. Dr. Brownstein shows why drugs have so many adverse effects. The following conditions are covered in this book: high cholesterol levels, depression, GERD and reflux esophagitis, osteoporosis, inflammation and hormone imbalances. He also gives examples of natural substances that can help the body heal.
See why the following drugs need to be avoided:

- Cholesterol-lowering drugs (statins such as Lipitor, Zocor, Mevacor, and Crestor)
- Antidepressant drugs (SSRI's such as Prozac, Zoloft, Celexa, Paxil)
- Antacid drugs (H-2 blockers and PPI's such as Nexium, Prilosec, and Zantac)
- Osteoporosis drugs (Bisphosphonates such as Fosomax and Actonel, Zometa, and Boniva)
- Anti-inflammatory drugs (Celebrex, Vioxx, Motrin, Naprosyn, etc)
- Synthetic Hormones (Provera and Estrogen)

SALT YOUR WAY TO HEALTH

Dr. Brownstein dispels many of the myths of salt. Salt is bad for you. Salt causes hypertension. These are just a few of the myths Dr. Brownstein tackles in this book. He shows you how the right kind of salt--unrefined salt--can have a remarkable health benefit to the body. Refined salt is a toxic, devitalized substance for the body. Unrefined salt is a necessary ingredient for achieving your optimal health. See how adding unrefined salt to your diet can help you:

- Maintain a normal blood pressure
- Balance your hormones
- Optimize your immune system
- Lower your risk for heart disease
- Overcome chronic illness
-

THE MIRACLE OF NATURAL HORMONES, 3RD EDITION

Optimal health cannot be achieved with an imbalanced hormonal system. Dr. Brownstein's research on bioidentical hormones provides the reader with a plethora of information on the benefits of balancing the hormonal system with bioidentical, natural hormones. This book is in its third edition. This book gives actual case studies of the benefits of natural hormones.

See how balancing the hormonal system can help:

- Arthritis and autoimmune disorders
- Chronic fatigue syndrome and fibromyalgia
- Heart disease
- Hypothyroidism
- Menopausal symptoms
- And much more!

THE GUIDE TO HEALTHY EATING

Which food do you buy? Where to shop? How do you prepare food? This book will answer all of these questions and much more. Dr. Brownstein co-wrote this book with his nutritionist, Sheryl Shenefelt, C.N. Eating the healthiest way is the most important thing you can do. This book contains recipes and information on how best to feed your family. See how eating a healthier diet can help you:

- Avoid chronic illness
- Enhance your immune system
- Improve your family's nutrition

THE GUIDE TO A GLUTEN-FREE DIET

What would you say if 16% of the population (1/6) had a serious, life-threatening illness that was only being diagnosed correctly only 3% of the time? Gluten-sensitivity is the most frequently missed diagnosis in the U.S. This book will show how you can incorporate a healthier lifestyle by becoming gluten-free.

- Why you should become gluten-free
- What illnesses are associated with gluten sensitivity
- How to shop and cook gluten-free
- Where to find gluten-free resources

Call 1-888-647-5616 or send a check or money order
Each Book $15!
Sales Tax: For Michigan residents, please add $.90 per book.

Shipping:		
	1-3 Books	$5.00
	4-5 Books:	$4.00
	6-7 Books:	$3.00
	8 Books: FREE SHIPPING!	

VOLUME DISCOUNTS AVAILABLE. CALL 1-888-647-5616 FOR MORE INFORMATION OR ORDER ON-LINE AT: WWW.DRBROWNSTEIN.COM

You can send a check to: Medical Alternatives Press
4173 Fieldbrook
West Bloomfield, MI 48323

Look at www.drbrownstein.com for more information on NEW DVD's of Dr. Brownstein's latest lectures and companion DVD's for each book!